THE
MILLIONAIRE'S
Diet

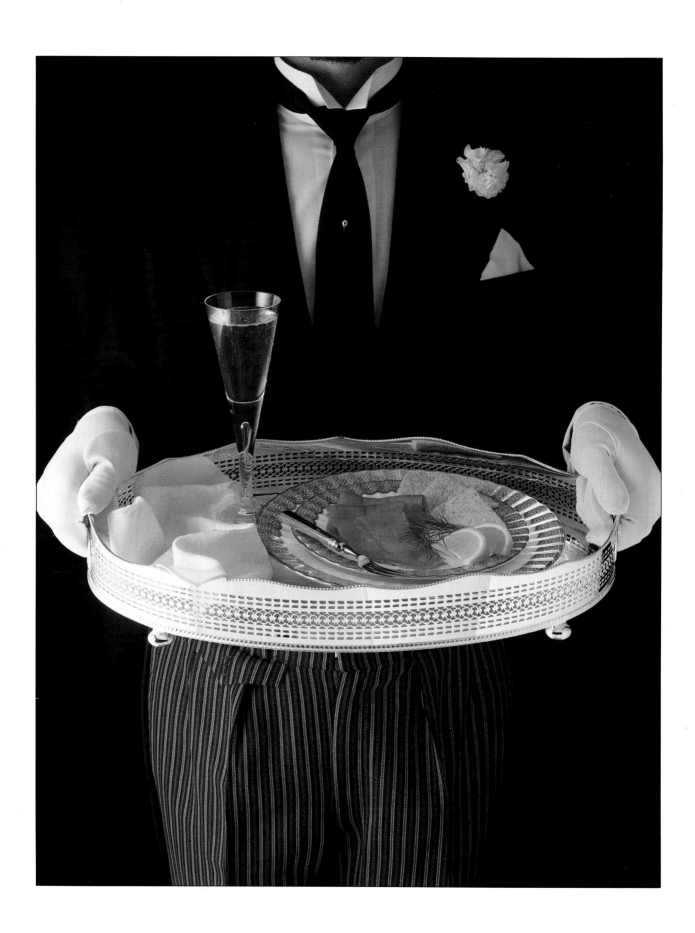

THE
MILLIONAIRE'S
Diet

LOYD GROSSMAN

Macdonald

A Macdonald BOOK

© Loyd Grossman 1985

First published in Great Britain in 1985
by Macdonald & Co (Publishers) Ltd
London & Sydney
A member of BPCC plc

British Library Cataloguing in Publication Data
Grossman, Loyd
   The millionaire's diet.
   1. Reducing diets—Recipes
   I. Title
   641.5′635   RM222.2

   ISBN 0-356-10869-4

Filmset by Text Filmsetters Limited, Orpington
Printed and bound in Great Britain by Purnell and Sons
(Book Production) Ltd, Paulton, Bristol
A member of BPCC plc

Editor: Barbara Horn
Designer: Richard Johnson
Assistant Designer: Clare Forte
Photographer: Clive Corless
Cover photographer: Peter Myers
Stylist: Dawn Lane
Home Economist: Michelle Thomson
The publishers wish to thank the
following organizations for the loan
of materials used in photography:
Cunard Line Ltd; Fortnum & Mason,
for briefcase, wines and food;
Hardy's of Pall Mall for fishing
and shooting equipment;
Lonsdale Sports Equipment Ltd,
for sports equipment;
Mappin & Webb, Regent Street, for
silver, glass and china;
Way In at Harrods.

Macdonald & Co (Publishers) Ltd
Maxwell House
74 Worship Street
London EC2A 2EN

CONTENTS

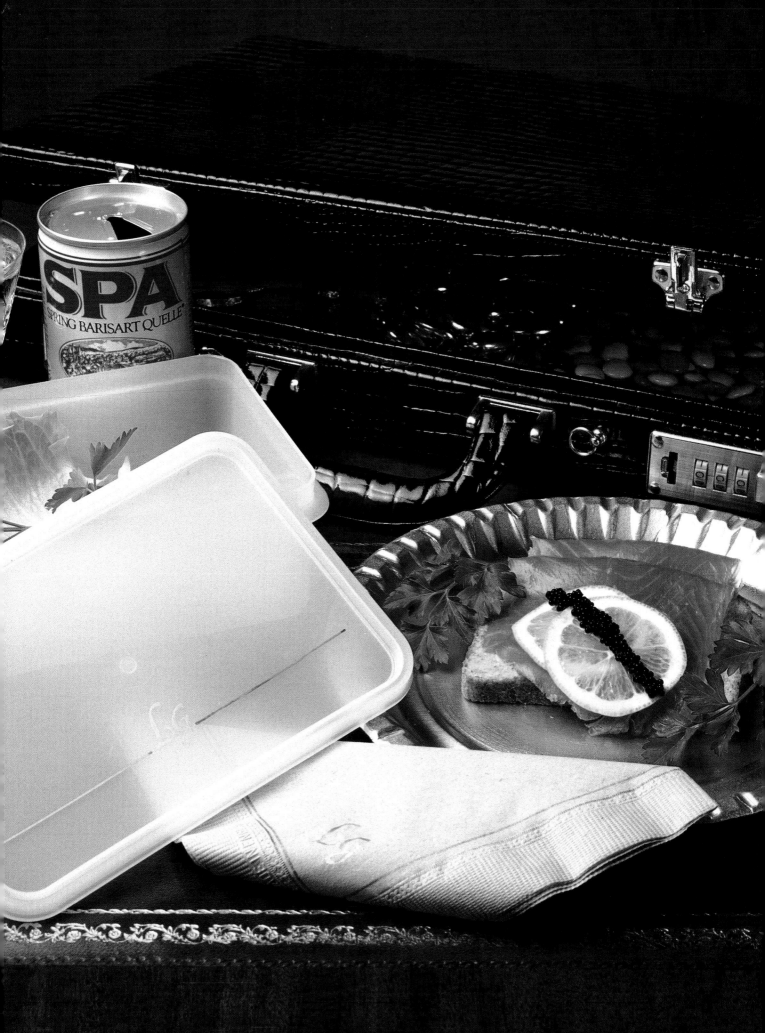

THE MILLIONAIRE'S DIET

This diet is not a course of punishment for being too fat—it is instead a luxurious low calorie regime. If you want to lose weight, you have to reduce calories, but you can do that without weeks of martyrdom through the medium of crispbread, diet margarine and undressed salad. Moderation and restraint aren't dirty or unpleasant words: what harm ever came from a small lobster or a half bottle of champagne?

Good plain food

In *Casino Royale* James Bond treated his companion to dinner at the Savoy. She ordered caviar, *rognons de veau*, *pommes soufflées* and *fraises des bois*, and turning to Bond asked 'Isn't it shameless to be so certain and so expensive?' 'It's a virtue', the gourmet spy replied 'and anyway it's good plain wholesome food.' Bond was perhaps slightly ahead of his time, as until very recently luxury was more likely to be associated with superabundance and baroque complexity rather than purity and simplicity.

The luxury foods of the rich have not remained constant. In a society where scarcity is the rule, abundance is the hallmark of the big-wig's dining table. Vitellius, least notable of the Roman emperors and classical glutton *par excellence* (when faced by a revolt of the Praetorian guards he fled with his cook and pastry cook), gave a banquet at which seven thousand game birds, two thousand fish, and bizarre concoctions of pike livers and flamingo tongues were served. In nineteenth-century Russia the aimless and wilfully perverse behaviour of the idle ruling class is well observed in Pushkin's description of Eugene Onegin's bachelor dinner:

'Before him roast beef red and gory,
and truffles which have ever been
youth's choice, the flower of French cuisine;
and pâté, Strasbourg's deathless glory,
sits with Limburg's vivacious cheese,
and *ananas* the gold of trees.
More wine he calls to drench
the fire of the cutlet's scalding fat.'

Few today could cope with a menu of pineapple, limburger, roast beef, veal cutlets and foie gras.

But even the rich must get back to basics: Aristotle Onassis's favourite dish was raw onions drenched in olive oil. Many of the foods that are considered the most extravagant – oysters, smoked salmon, game – are the purest and the best. Joe Public may think that good plain food is a steak-and-kidney pudding with marrowfat peas – *we* know that he's romanticizing trash. Our plate of asparagus followed by a roast partridge is what wholesome food is meant to be.

Those of us who are middle middle class and above tend to eat and drink far too much. In upmarket lives the social role of eating is so important (we talk at table) that as many as five hours a day are spent eating and drinking. It would be foolish and damned unpleasant to give up business lunches, drinks parties and dinners, but we must do something to stop looking like the Michelin man. Exercise, as is reasonably well known, is not enough; indeed exercise alone will do almost nothing. (What it *will* do is help you to give up some of your worst habits. There's nothing more agonizing than having to bicycle to work the morning after you've drunk eleven Pimms and smoked a pack and a half of Marlboroughs.) With this diet all you need is a certain measure of discipline; there are enough treats to mitigate the chore of self-control.

Nonetheless there is an enormous list of absolute no-nos, Forbidden Foods whose denial may irritate you more than slightly. But if you're to lose any weight at all, you'll have to go without . . . without mayonnaise, pudding, pastry, bread and butter, cream, biscuits, spirits, bacon, sausages, mashed potatoes, jam, marmalade, port, crisps and nuts, just to begin the list. Actually, it's not quite as prohibitive as it seems: we do become habituated to eating an awful lot of stuff that is neither particularly good for us, nor, for that matter, particularly tasty.

In 1650 Thomas Moffat wrote that

'There be two vices, Surfeiting when a man eateth
More than either his Stomach can hold or his Strength
digest and self-pining when we eat less than our
Nature craveth and is able to overcome.'

The difficulty is, of course, in striking a balance: enough may be as good as the proverbial feast, but what is enough?

Ideas of enough have varied considerably, and it's instructive to look at the diet of Mr Banting, whose continual efforts to reduce his gargantuan girth gave us a once popular slang word for dieting: banting.

Breakfast

6 oz boiled fish
Slice dry toast
Large coffee

Lunch

6 oz boiled fish
Any vegetable (excepting potatoes or carrots)
Any fruit
6 oz game
3 glasses of claret

Tea

3 oz cooked fruit
A rusk
Black tea

Supper

4 oz meat or fish
2 glasses claret

Nightcap

2 glasses claret

Unlike Mr Banting's binge the method of this diet is to limit daily intake to about 1500 calories. Calories may be the crudest measure of whether a food is likely to be fattening – there have been carbohydrate, protein and fibre based diets – but on balance it seems that calories provide the most reasonable guide to what and how much we can eat. Most of the breakfast and lunch menus are intended for one person eating alone, while all the dinners are designed for two to enjoy together.

JUST A LITTLE DRINK

Alcohol, alas is appallingly fattening as well as being a menace to life, liver and memory. It is impossible to lose weight without substantially reducing alcohol intake, although, thankfully, it need not be given up altogether. If you find even limiting your drink so very difficult you could try surviving on two bottles of Margaux and a pound of raw carrots a day, or adopt the F. Scott Fitzgerald diet of two dozen bottles of beer and no food, alternated with Coca-Cola and coffee days or bottle-of-gin and intravenous glucose days, but we don't recommend any of it. Not only will you not lose any weight (alcohol deadens self-control and after the first bottle of wine you could actually swallow half a Gâteau St Honoré before you even remembered that you were supposed to be on a diet), but also you will certainly lose what good looks you have, a lot of money and a good many friends.

Abstaining from drink might indeed be the best thing to do, but it really is asking too much. In any event a *moderate* intake of alcohol is meant to help our digestion and may even help us to live longer. This diet renounces spirits—far more calorific than wine—and recommends a paltry half bottle of wine a day, which may barely slake the parched plutocrat's thirst, but still is just enough to make the world seem a slightly better place. Dry wine is, of course, less fattening

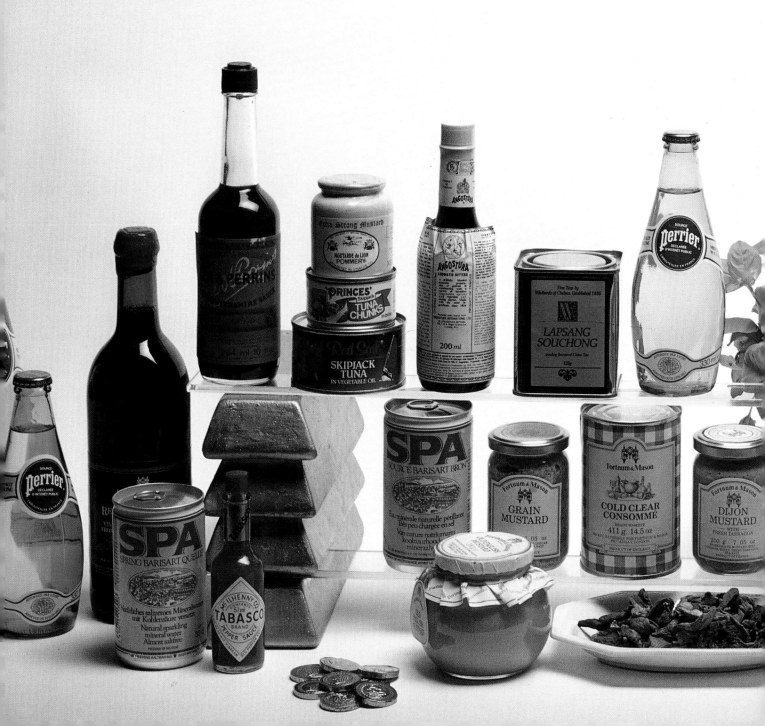

than sweet wine, white less fattening than red, although the difference between dry white and red is a mere 5 calories a glass.

TAKING THE WATERS

Solace may now be found in the large range of mineral waters quite readily available, and it is wonderful how an absence of alcohol concentrates the mind on the differences in taste produced by the presence of lesser or greater amounts of potassium or silica. In some forms this much despised beverage, normally thought of as useful only for shaving or boiling asparagus, can be both delicious and

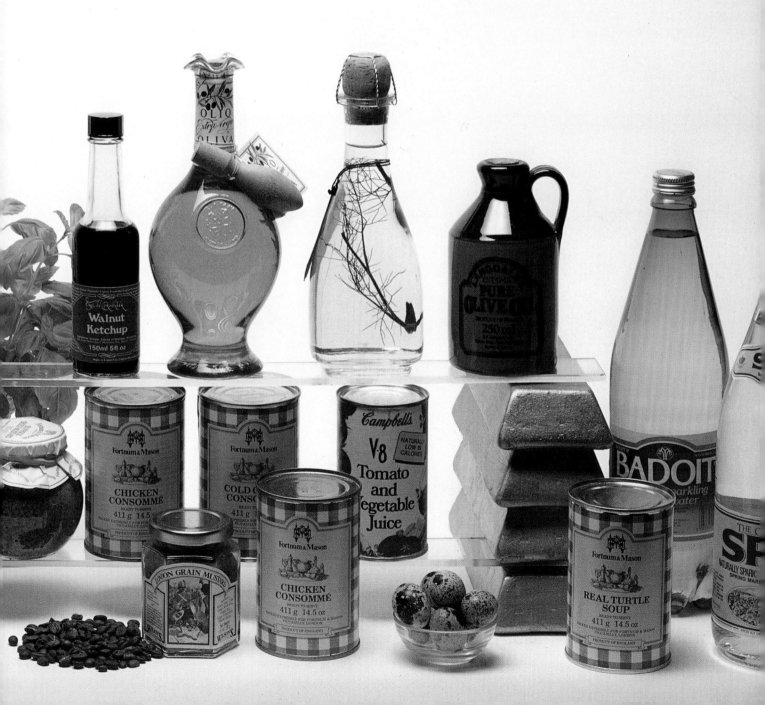

refreshing. True connoisseurs of bottled water are most fond of Italian waters with their clearly labelled mineral composition certified by undistinguished professors of hydrotherapy at obscure provincial universities. French waters tend to be cagey about their constituents while unspeakably *nouveau* English waters blind the drinker with historical claptrap about Roman encampments, druidic springs and the like.

Perrier, unquestionably the most fashionable water thanks to its splendid bottle and marvellous advertising, is for many overgassified. Source Badoit is much more distinguished, but many people find it slightly sweet and perhaps too reticent in its carbonation. The same may be said about San Pellegrino, although my feeling is that it is the most elegant and drinkable of all waters. The northern waters of Spa and Apollinaris are perfectly all right, if rather bland and conservative. Many of the English supermarket waters are, like Perrier, too obviously sparkling — handy if you've left them overnight but after two glasses you feel like the Goodyear blimp. I have never been a partisan of still waters — quite frankly they are not sufficiently different from tap water to be at all interesting. The great exception must be the extremely alkaline Vichy, which really ought not to be drunk with food at all — it tastes too much as if you've left washing-up liquid on your fork.

Desperate drinkers and fantasists may add as much water as they like to their wine: sometimes an illusion of quantity may be comforting. Fresh fruit juices are healthy but unexciting. The best emergency drink to take your mind off all those missed cocktails is a stiff Virgin Mary (sometimes more evocatively known as a Bloody Shame), far more therapeutic in the making and restorative in the drinking than a mere tarted-up glass of tomato juice. Begin with about 8 fl oz (240 ml) of chilled tomato or, preferably, V-8 juice, a blended vegetable juice. (Other blended vegetable juices vary tremendously: Lindavia is acceptable, Epicure isn't). Add the juice of at least one half lemon, or, if feeling in need of serious revivification, one whole lemon. Most Virgin and Bloody Marys suffer outrageously from too liberal dosing of Worcestershire and Tabasco sauces. Shake in just four or five drops of Worcestershire — after all, you're not some ignorant bartender — then possibly three drops of Tabasco. Remember that tabasco is mostly vinegar and too much will be absolutely disgusting. I sometimes prefer to use other hot sauces, such as the luridly green Bruce's Tango Sauce or the milder, popular Brazilian brand, Cica. Sometimes it is best to dispense with Tabasco and its brothers completely and merely add a teaspoon of prepared horseradish. Horseradish gives a greatly superior burn, but if used the drink has to be made in a cocktail shaker and strained to avoid frog-spawn-like globules. Finally, add either a rib of celery (some perverts prefer a stick of cucumber) or some celery salt and a few good grinds of black pepper. You won't miss the vodka.

TEA AND COFFEE

Vital but unexciting, tea and coffee may be drunk freely provided you don't add milk and sugar. Beware of too much coffee – severe shakes will not help your diet or temper. The strong and tarry Lapsang Souchong is particularly good unadorned, as are strongly scented teas like Earl Grey and Russian Caravan.

OIL AND VINEGAR

Oil, it must be said, at 132 calories a tablespoon is not a normal part of most diets. But if you're going to eat salads (and you *are* going to) oil is indispensable. Olive oil is the top oil, but a good walnut or hazlenut oil is also worth using for the sake of variety. Corn oil, peanut oil and 'salad oil' do not exist for the purposes of good eating and anyone who uses them on a salad should be flung into prison.

There are countless olive oils available and even the most ordinary is far superior to other types of oil. The finest oils (that is, those with the lowest acidity) are the so-called extra virgin oils. Both France and Italy produce very fine oils and whether one wants a pale and delicate light oil or something darker and a bit more assertive is a matter of personal taste. Top oils are nightmarishly expensive (only your account will notice) and well worth it. Cheap and nondescript Spanish and Greek oils can be given a miss. Although there are some very distinguished Greek oils, few of them are exported in any quantity, but the search for interesting oils may add variety to an otherwise boring Aegean yachting holiday.

After oil, the most important salad ingredient is vinegar (lemon is a worthy substitute only in a few specific salads, such as Caesar Salad). In general the trendy obsession with strawberry and other absurdly flavoured vinegars is of little relevance to salad making. Malt vinegar is anathema – only wine vinegar can be used on a salad, and its quality makes the greatest difference. There are smart French vinegars (the most readily available come in tall stoneware crocks like geneva bottles) but by far the best vinegars are Italian, some so pure and delicious that you can drink them. My own favourites are the *aceti balsamicos* (balsam vinegars) produced around Modena, which add an incomparable flavour to most salads (although you must not use them on Salade Niçoise). Balsamico is not cheap: like fine wine, it is produced in vintages and is said to be better after fifty years in the bottle.

After insuring the absolute superiority of your ingredients, good taste rather than genius is the only insurance for a good salad

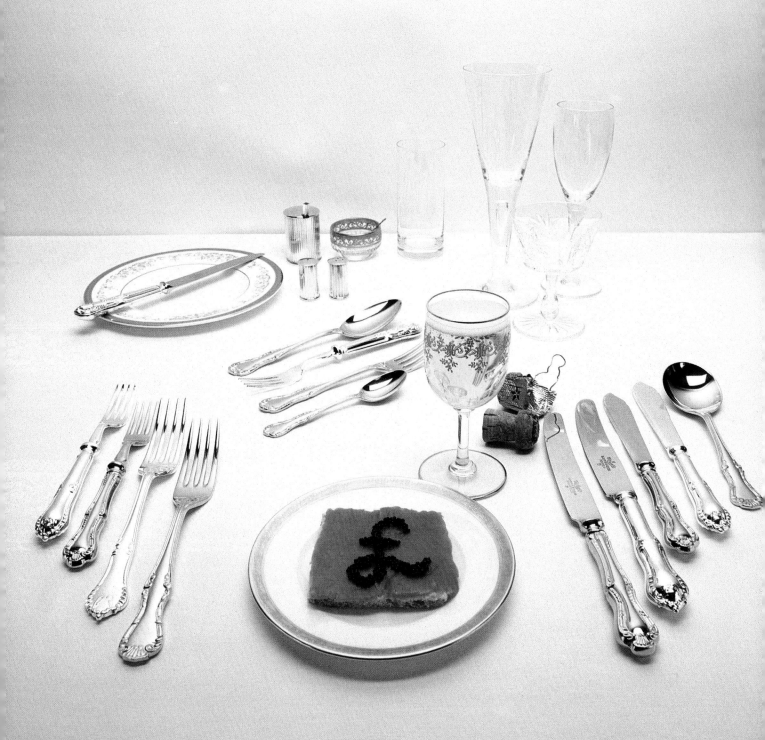

dressing. There are endless Mediterranean folk aphorisms about being a spendthrift with oil, a miser with vinegar, a philosopher with salt, and so on. Simply remember to exercise extreme discretion with the vinegar and avoid the addition of any superfluous ingredients like Worcestershire sauce, cream, or pink peppercorns. For slight variations you might want to add some finely chopped fresh basil or chervil, or perhaps steep a clove of garlic in the oil for a few hours. The most important codicil to any advice on salad dressings is to be sure and toss the salad properly to insure a very light but even coating and no oil slick at the bottom. Buy the biggest bowl you can afford – and with your money it should be huge.

EATING OUT

The minefield of restaurant lunches and dinner parties must be crossed by any would be successful dieter. Dinner parties are most perilous, as the temptation and sometimes even the necessity to overeat and drink are ominously present. Lashings of Perrier cannot ease the boredom of being seated next to a woman from Esher or a Swindonian chartered accountant. If you are presented with a dinner of delicatessen *pâté de campagne*, overwrought lasagne and recently defrosted Blackforest Cake, your diet could be set back for a week. So during the diet the best course of action is to turn down invitations from all but the closest friends and shamelessly forbid them to press Beef Wellington or Lobster Thermidor on you. Keep on the water, avoid second helpings and take as much salad as possible: you will survive. Better yet, try to stay at home.

Restaurant meals are much less difficult. Avoid Indian restaurants, where food tends to be swimming in lurid orange oil or else bathed in unidentifiable creamy substances. If you're absolutely gasping for heat and dust, restrict yourself to the plainest dishes like tandoori chicken or lobster, which sprinkled with lemon juice and served with salad make a perfectly acceptable lunch. French restaurants will usually offer one or two plain dishes, such as a *poule au pot* or a poached fish, but you must shun any heavily sauced dishes and calorifically lethal first courses like terrines or anything whose success depends on an accompaniment of endless buttered toast. So-called *nouvelle cuisine* – more accurately *nouvellesque* – restaurants, are most difficult – too often in Britain this sort of cookery is merely a trendy farrago of inept technique and inconceivably uncomfortable combinations of ingredients. Italian restaurants – good Italian restaurants that is – are frightfully good for people on diets as long as you avoid heavily sauced pastas. Trattorias generally offer the largest range of healthful Western European food and are most accommodating about making up large salads or plates of well-arranged properly cooked vegetables. The minimalist nature of Japanese cuisine makes it ideal for any weight-watcher so long as you don't order any fried dishes. Chinese restaurants may be more of a problem, as less distinguished Chinese cooks like to drown their vegetables in sauces that have been too boldly thickened with cornflour and laced with palate-slaying quantities of MSG (monosodium glutamate).

When ordering in any restaurant, follow the general precepts of the diet. Prefer fish, chicken or turkey to meat; favour poached, grilled or baked foods to sautéd or fried; dress your own salad; and ask for vegetables to be unbuttered. If faced with an array of fatty, creamy or buttery first courses, ask for, say, a tomato and onion salad or a plate of smoked salmon. Fruit (fresh and whole, not in fruit salad) is the only acceptable dessert, but if you haven't drunk any wine, you are allowed to treat yourself to a small sorbet or ice cream. Fortunately, most restaurants will be able to give you a plain grilled sole, although this poor fish is too often used as a mere sponge for butter. Sadly, the quality of salads and vegetables — with the exception of absolutely prohibited food like chips and *pommes dauphinoise* — in most restaurants is abysmal. But with restaurants, as with life, the more you care to spend, the more likely you are to get what you want, and most plutocratic feeding stations will gladly supply you with half a dozen oysters followed by a little poached salmon and a reasonable green salad.

Never eat on a train, a cross channel ferry or a plane unless you have ordered a special meal in advance. Feeling sick and getting fat at the same time is not on. If you are rich enough to be reading this book, you will probably never go into a transport cafe, where everything is fatty, fried or otherwise horrible. If you can possibly cut down on the number of your business lunches, do so. Eating at your desk means that you won't be so tempted to drink. Still it may be wise to lock the desk drawer where you store your whisky and give the key to your secretary. Sandwich-bar salads tend to be too enthusiastically dressed or salad-creamed, but such places are generally willing to supply you with a plate of turkey or possibly a double thickness smoked salmon sandwich (discard the top slice of bread). It is possible to have a small tub of cottage cheese and a sliced tomato, but awfully depressing. Not lunching out may cause a drastic rise in your productivity and efficiency, which will be almost impossible to sustain when you return to your old business lunch habits. So if lunching in, spend at least one and a half hours reading some form of light thriller or devote the same amount of time to shopping or museum going.

BREAKFAST BRIEF

All nutritionists stress the importance of a good breakfast as part of any dietary regime. We all know that breakfast is good for us — it prevents mid-morning fatigue and keeps us from overeating later in the day — but most breakfasts are just a bore. Breakfast ought to consist of kedgeree, brioches, grilled kidneys, and Haddock Monte Carlo consumed in vast quantities and at great leisure to the accompaniment of rustling newspapers. Such breakfasts are not made for busy people on working days and even minor league millionaires will be far too busy with the press, the post and the demands of the new day to devote the proper time and attention to it. The breakfast of quickly knocked up scrambled eggs, two slices of buttered tasteless toast and milky instant coffee is both unsatisfying and undesirable.

A glass of freshly squeezed (never ever out of a carton) orange juice — perhaps spiked with a few drops of angostura bitters, or grapefruit juice — squeezed the night before and infused overnight with a few mint leaves is indispensable at the start of the day, and followed by unsweetened black tea or coffee ought to be enough to get one going. The whole idea of health drinks, (those turgid commercial concoctions spiked with enough vitamins to last you a year) is deplorable: try a glass of sweetened Indian lassee instead. Perhaps the best low-calorie breakfast is a peach or pear accompanied by some well-chilled yoghurt. Greek yoghurt is by far the best, but there are some good live English ones. Breakfasts have been included in the book for those with the discipline, desire or desperation to have them.

SNACKING

Everyone gets hungry between meals. Diets often tell you that you can have an unlimited quantity of rabbit food to fill the gaps in the day, but who wants a celery stick at 4:30? Unfortunately, most of the snacks that hard core snackers like aren't really allowed — one Mars bar can sink a whole week of sensible eating. The only acceptable snacks really are rabbit food, fresh (definitely not dried) fruit and clear soups like turtle soup with a teaspoon of very dry sherry or Madeira, and beef consommé, which is excellent chilled.

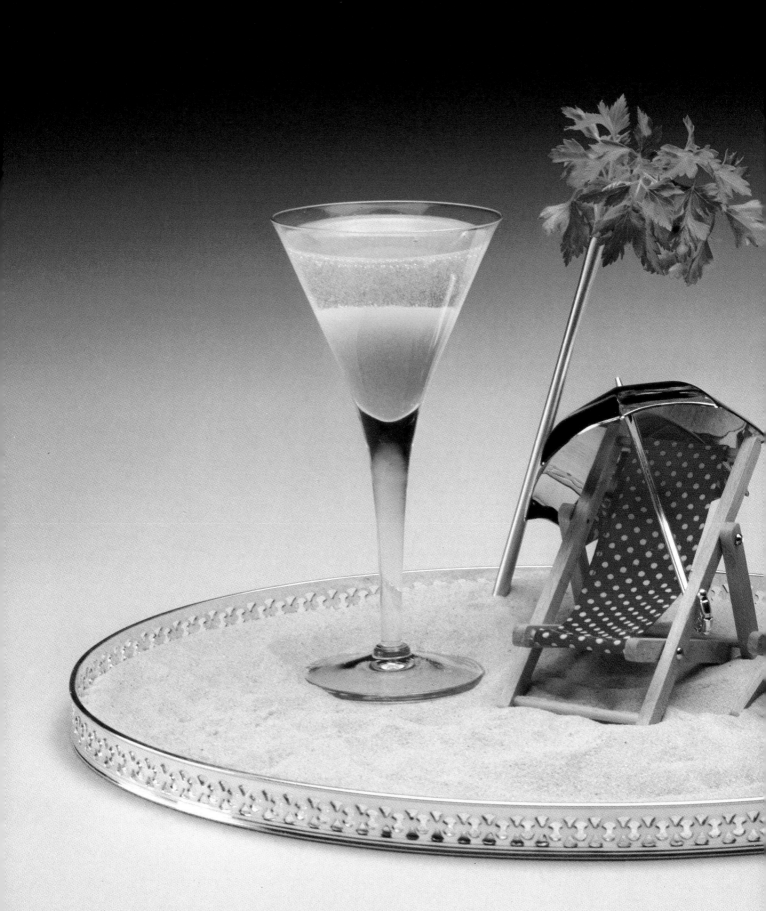

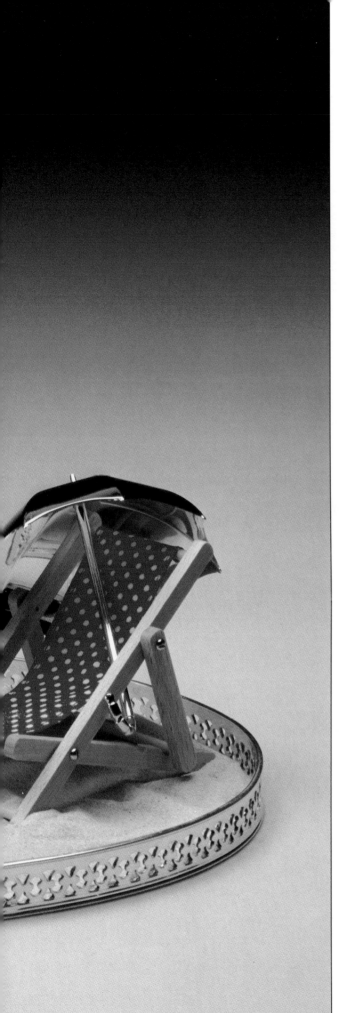

DAY 1

FRENCH RIVIERA DAY

As the French Riviera becomes increasingly populated by brigands and the lower middle classes, the fleeting joys of the SOF may be more satisfactorily evoked in the kitchen.

BREAKFAST

1 Mango Bellini
1 soft-boiled duck egg
Crispbread
Lapsang Souchong tea

To make the Mango Bellini put 2 tablespoons mango purée in a tall glass. Top up with champagne (not some cheap sparkler – you can tell the difference *even* in mixed drinks). Stir well. Crispbread, in most cases unfortunately reminiscent of roofing insulation, has been developed to its highest form by the Scandinavians. There are thin wafer-like crispbreads and great hulking wheels of the stuff. The easiest to cope with is probably one of the very high fibre varieties. (But you must enjoy chewing. As you slowly work your way through a slab remember that Avicenna counselled sixty chews per mouthful.)

Drink the tea very hot, not too strong, and without any additives. A thin slice of lemon may be allowed if you are not a connoisseur.

LUNCH

If taken in the office

1 open-faced smoked salmon sandwich, on
plain brown bread with a wedge of lemon.
As much mineral water as you like. The
harder, fizzier waters are best with fish.

In a restaurant

Tomato and onion salad
Grilled fillet steak
Plain boiled spinach

DINNER

If you have had a reasonably substantial restaurant lunch or a high protein sandwich, a salad-based dinner is most appropriate.

Salade Niçoise is one of the most travestied classic dishes, often appearing as a preposterous dumping ground for stray odds and ends from the kitchen – I have even been served one containing canned sweetcorn! The canonical Niçoise as recorded by Jaques Medecin in *Cuisine Niçoise* is far more rigorous than most more familiar versions. Medecin calls for salted quartered tomatoes, hard-boiled eggs, anchovy or tuna (not both), cucumber, green pepper, spring onions, olives, broad beans or artichokes, and basil.

I prefer a slightly more relaxed version. Remember when making this or any other salad to use the largest bowl you have – the more space you have for tossing the salad, the less dressing you will need. Remember, too, that a dressing is meant to *lightly* cover the contents of the salad.

Salad Niçoise

4 tomatoes
½ large cucumber
1 green pepper
7 oz/200 g can tuna fish in brine
2 hard-boiled eggs
8 oz/225 g lightly cooked french beans
6 fat black olives
8 anchovy fillets
3 large leaves fresh basil
4 tbsp olive oil
¼ lemon

Core and quarter the tomatoes. Peel the cucumber and slice it thinly. Slice the green pepper into thin strips. Drain the tuna and shred it with a fork. Shell and quarter the hard-boiled eggs. Combine in a large bowl, then add the cold french beans, olives and anchovy fillets. Tear the basil leaves in your fingers and add to the salad. (Never cut basil with steel, as it stains the herb and may also affect the taste.) Pour the olive oil onto the salad and squeeze the lemon over it. Toss the salad thoroughly, but not violently. Chill for 30 minutes.

You may have half a bottle of cheap white wine, such as a Gros Plant, with this, as the salad's strong flavours aren't particularly kind to important wines.

DAY 2

GREEK TYCOON'S DAY

We've seen that Onassis adored raw onions and oil, but that's no reason for you to let the side down. Enjoy a high-protein lunch and dinner, and you might even forget you are on a diet.

BREAKFAST

Glass of fresh orange juice
½ pot Greek yoghurt
1 banana
Unsweetened black tea or coffee

More violence is done to yoghurt than to most foods. It is oversweet or oversour or overthickened or just otherwise repellent. Most people shy away from the stuff after suffering at the pots of supermarket varieties with jocular continental names. The best Greek yoghurt is refreshing, well balanced, and utterly delicious, although those whose palates have been mugged by a lifelong addiction to Mars bars may still wish to sweeten it ever so slightly with perhaps a teaspoon of honey (Greek, of course). If unable to find the real thing (now fairly well distributed), some English boutique brands (Loseley for instance) are perfectly acceptable.

LUNCH

Mixed salad (as a first course)
Grilled noisette of lamb
Broccoli

DINNER

Fish soup
Granita

There are endless but not dissimilar variations on a basic fish soup, all involving lightly sautéing a mixture of aromatic vegetables (such as celery, leek and onion), then adding fish and simmering the lot in water, stock or wine with the occasional addition of milk, cream or tomatoes. This fish soup is actually more of a stew and a distant cousin to New England fish chowder.

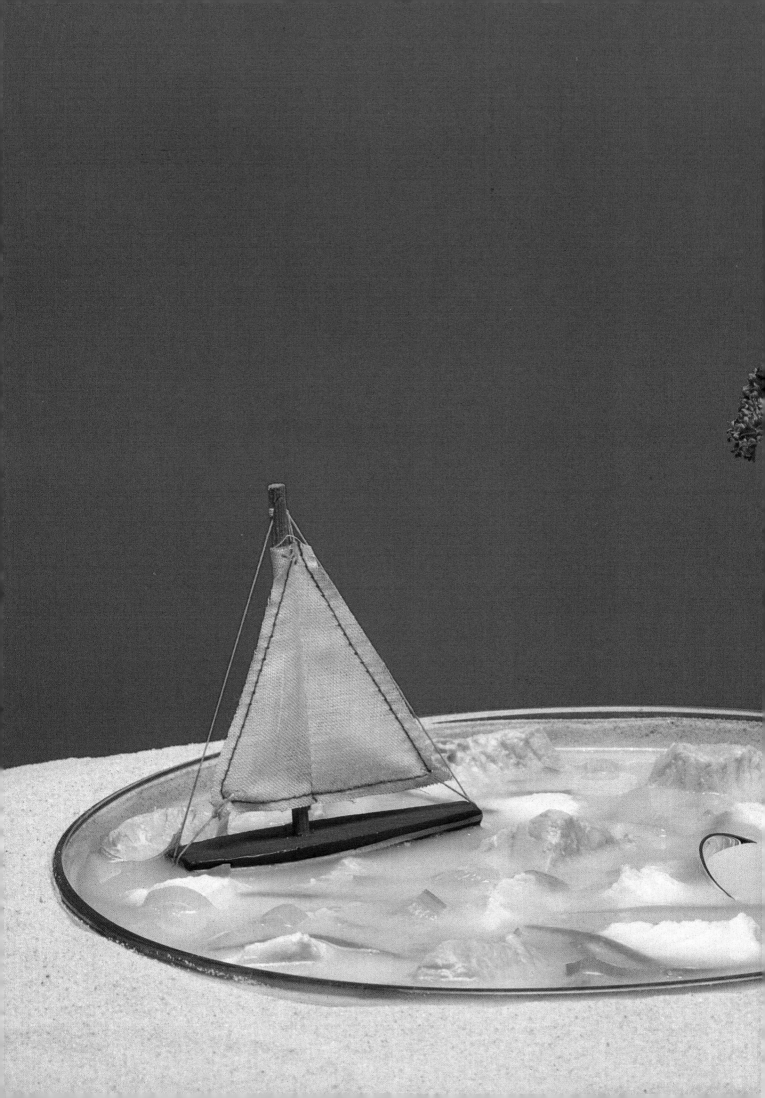

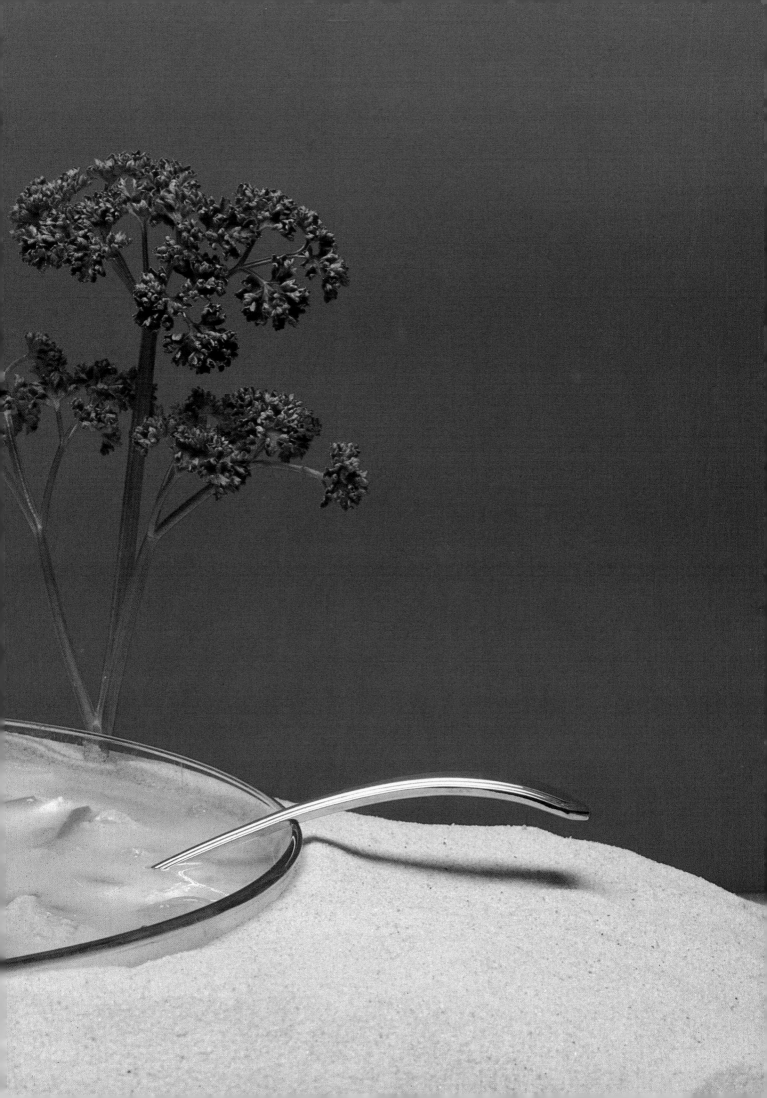

Fish soup

4 carrots
2 sticks celery
2 leeks
1½ oz/40g butter
1 large salmon steak, skinned and cubed
1 large halibut steak, skinned and cubed
4 large scallops without the coral
fish stock or water
dry white wine
fresh chopped chives or basil

Julienne the carrots and chop the celery and leeks into small pieces. Melt the butter in a heavy saucepan and slowly cook the vegetables so that they begin to soften but do not brown; if they show signs of browning, lower the heat. Add the salmon and halibut pieces and cook slowly until they begin to turn opaque and lose their 'raw' colour. Add the scallops. When they too have lost their raw colour, cover with the stock and white wine, bring to the boil and then simmer slowly for about 20 minutes. Just before serving, garnish with chopped chives or basil.

For a rather more Greek flavoured fish soup use 1 tablespoon oil instead of butter and a handful of chopped celery leaves instead of the leeks.

A good Sancerre goes well with this. For non-drinkers the meal can be accompanied by some boiled orzo (a Greek pasta shaped like grains of rice) or a few new potatoes.

Granita

If by now you're absolutely *dying* for a pudding, you have suffered enough and may console yourself with some granita, an Italian ice that even Greek tycoons consider a treat. The best granita is coffee, and the best coffee granita is this one from Marcella Hazsan's wonderfully good *Classic Italian Cooking*.

2 tbsp caster sugar
¾ pint/450 ml cold espresso

Dissolve the sugar in the cold espresso. Pour the mixture into two freezer trays and place in the freezer for 15 minutes. Remove and stir to break up the ice. Return to the freezer for 15 minutes; remove and stir again. Return to the freezer for 10 minutes; remove and stir. Return to the freezer for 8 minutes; remove and stir. Then return to the freezer and stir the coffee every 8 minutes for 3 hours. This, it must be said, is extremely tiresome and only for those who *must* have some pudding that isn't fruit, and have a servant who can be spared to do nothing else.

DAY 3

PLUTOCRAT'S PICNIC DAY

If properly carried off, this should nicely re-create the joys of extremely expensive cold food consumed in luxurious, through slightly rough and ready, surroundings. Bring a cashmere rug to the office with you, spread it on the floor, sit down and munch.

BREAKFAST

Glass of fresh orange juice
½ pot yoghurt
1 pear
Unsweetened black tea or coffee

LUNCH

It's about time to have lunch in the office. Do not send your secretary to the local sarni bar for liverwurst on white – this is a day for serious brownbagging. You can bring all the essential elements to the office with you in the Plutocrat's Lunch Box, but the final assembly must take place just before you eat. Buy a metal briefcase – there are a large number of Italian ones that can be kept in the fridge. Pack the following ingredients for one, as well as a knife, spoons and tableware.

1 ripe avocado
2oz/50g salmon caviar
1 lemon
1 ripe peach
1 miniature bottle brandy
2 small bottles mineral water

The excessively lazy may be tempted to let a servant prepare their avocado in the morning, but by lunchtime it will be a rather unpleasant brown. If you want to avoid having sharp knives in the office (most dangerous in the case of staff discontent), salad avocados are an amusing alternative – small and stoneless, they are eaten skin and all, but must be very ripe. Indeed, the issue of avocado ripeness is most problematical, as the underripe are disgusting and almost inedible, and the overripe are mushy and unappealing. One of the most practical skills anyone can have is the ability to tell a ripe avo by feel – only experience can teach. The hamhanded must consign their fate to an honest greengrocer.

Cut the avocado in half, remove the stone and stuff each hollow with half the salmon caviar. Dress with a squeeze of lemon. Skin, stone and slice the peach and pour a tablespoon of brandy over it. Drink the water, perhaps Ramlosa in this case, with the meal – but don't let the rest of the brandy go to waste; a millionaire need not squander.

DINNER

Dried duck salad

Duck is frightfully fattening, especially because the rich and crispy skin of well-roasted duck is irresistible. Dried duck is a good way to satisfy one's craving and makes a particularly good salad. Be sure to remove all the extraneous fat from the duck.

7 oz/200g dried duck breast
1 head of radicchio
1 head curly endive
6 quail's eggs
3 tbsp olive oil
1 tbsp balsam vinegar

Trim all the fat from the duck and cut into bite-sized pieces. Remove any unattractive outside leaves from the radicchio, rinse the remaining leaves well and dry in a salad spinner, then either shred or tear them into pieces. Tear the curly endive into separate leaves, rinse and dry. Hard boil the quail's eggs by placing them in a pan of cold water and bringing to the boil. Then run cold water over the eggs and begin the incredibly irritating task of peeling the little brutes.

Salads made from ingredients like this rather unfortunately lend themselves to over-elaborate decoration, but I find this interior decorator style of cooking at home remarkably pretentious. So, unless you are a thwarted chintz merchant, place all the ingredients into a huge bowl, add the olive oil and vinegar and toss thoroughly.

This is very well accompanied by a half bottle of a superior Gewürztraminer.

For pudding, a small dish of *fraises des bois* seasoned with a few grinds of black pepper or a few squeezes of half an orange.

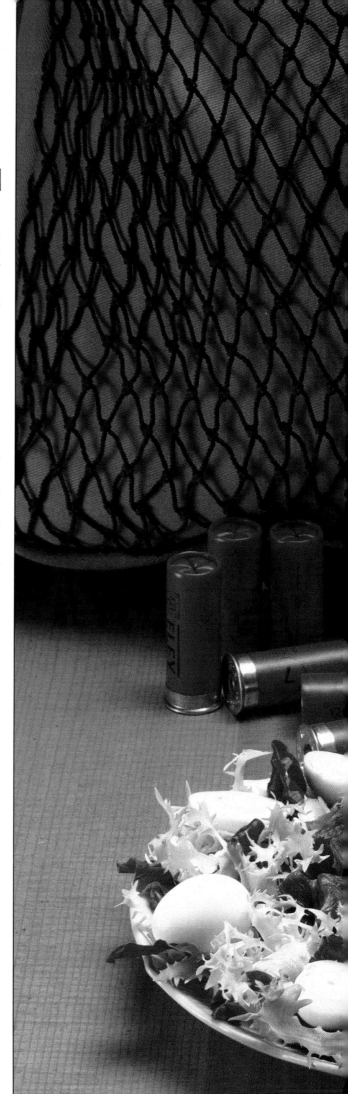

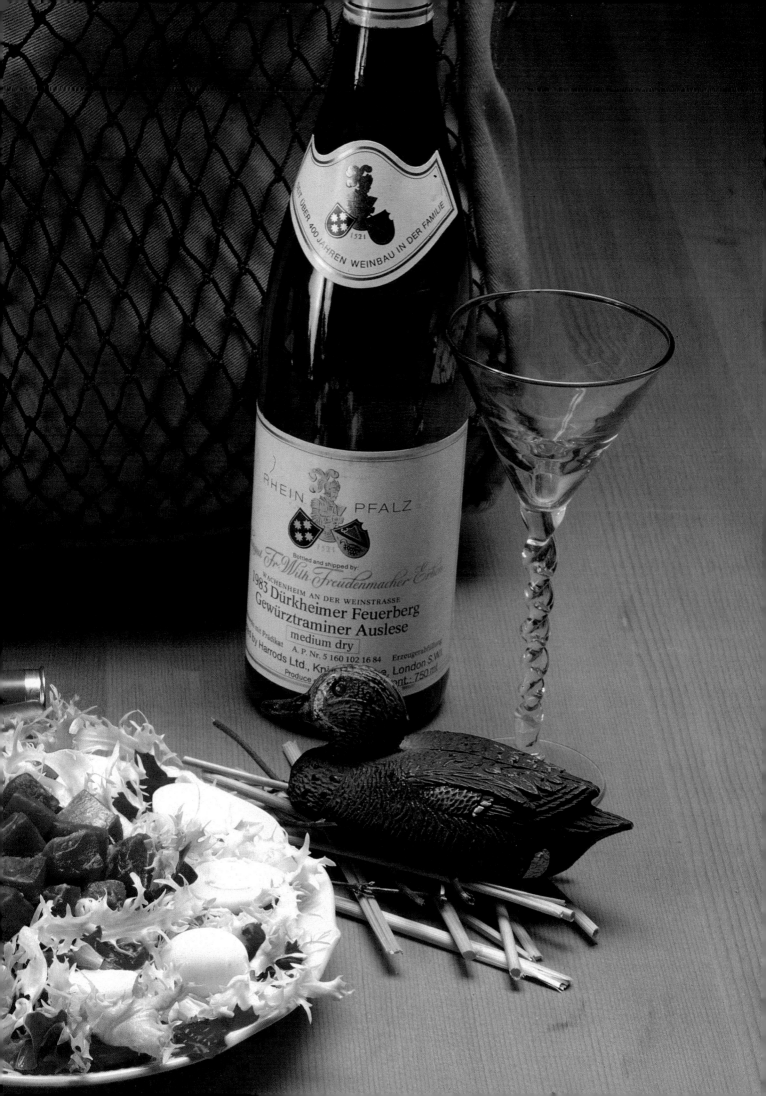

DAY 4

INTELLECTUAL'S DAY

There is no demonstrable causal connection between brains and money, but just in case...

BREAKFAST

½ grapefruit
1 tbsp comb honey
1 tsp fresh chopped ginger
1 slice wholemeal bread
Unsweetened black tea or coffee

Just to make sure your brain has started to function, you mix the honey with the ginger, then spread it on the bread. The real test is to see if you can eat it without getting sticky fingers.

LUNCH

Unusually for a seventeenth-century Englishman, Sir Isaac Newton had a passion for salads. Newton probably ate some form of salmagundi – the incredibly elaborate and to modern tastes vaguely unpalatable composed salad of Renaissance England. This slightly fanciful Salad Newton is more attuned to twentieth-century philosophers.

Salad Newton

4oz/100g raw spinach
4oz/100g smoked chicken
1 ripe avocado
2 spring onions
8 hard-boiled quail's eggs
3 tbsp walnut oil
1 tbsp balsam vinegar
salt and pepper

Wash the spinach and remove the stalks. Shred the smoked chicken, slice the avocado, and finely chop the spring onions. Combine in a large bowl with the quail's eggs, and dress with the oil and vinegar. Season with salt and black pepper.

Enjoy with a glass or two of the best mineral water.

DINNER

Classic brainfood
Peas and spinach purée
Pastiche Melba

Outside of Mediterranean Europe and Japan, fresh tuna is preposterously underrated. Perhaps some people find its beef-like appearance off-putting. Consequently it isn't very easy to get, but it should be sought out sedulously. A ravishing tuna stew is made around St Jean de Luz, but the best tuna I have ever had was simply grilled in Greece.

Classic brainfood

2 tuna steaks
olive oil
flour
oregano
freshly squeezed lime juice
black pepper

If all your fishmonger has is frozen tuna, make do with it — you'll still enjoy the treat. Heat a cast-iron grill or frying pan until it is very hot, then reduce heat to medium. Lightly smear the tuna steaks with a strongly flavoured olive oil, dust gently with flour and season with oregano. Put on the grill and turn over after about 5 minutes. A further 5 minutes should cook the tuna through. You will notice that as the tuna cooks, it turns a tan colour rather like canned tuna. Be sure to cook it through, but not to overcook it, as tuna tends to be a bit dry. Remove to a hot plate and season liberally with the freshly squeezed lime juice and black pepper.

Pear and spinach purée

Most purées rely far too heavily on butter or cream to be much use to us, but this refreshingly original recipe from Michel Guerard's *Cuisine Minceur* is both light and unusual.

2 oz/50 g pears
7 oz/200 g raw spinach
black pepper

Peel, quarter and core the pears and boil them for 15 minutes. Wash the spinach, remove the stalks and cook in boiling salted water for 3 minutes. Purée the spinach and pears in a food processor and season with black pepper. It's delicious, and not as fanciful as it sounds.

Pastiche Melba

5 oz/140 g fresh raspberries
2 ripe peaches

This is, alas, not Peach Melba as Escoffier intended, but a fair pastiche that avoids any added sugar.
  Purée the raspberries in a food processor. Stone and peel the peaches and cut each into eighths. Arrange the peach slices artistically, if you're so inclined, and pour the raspberry purée over them. This might have helped Nellie keep her figure.
  A decent white Mâcon goes quite well with this meal, as does a large bottle of mineral water.

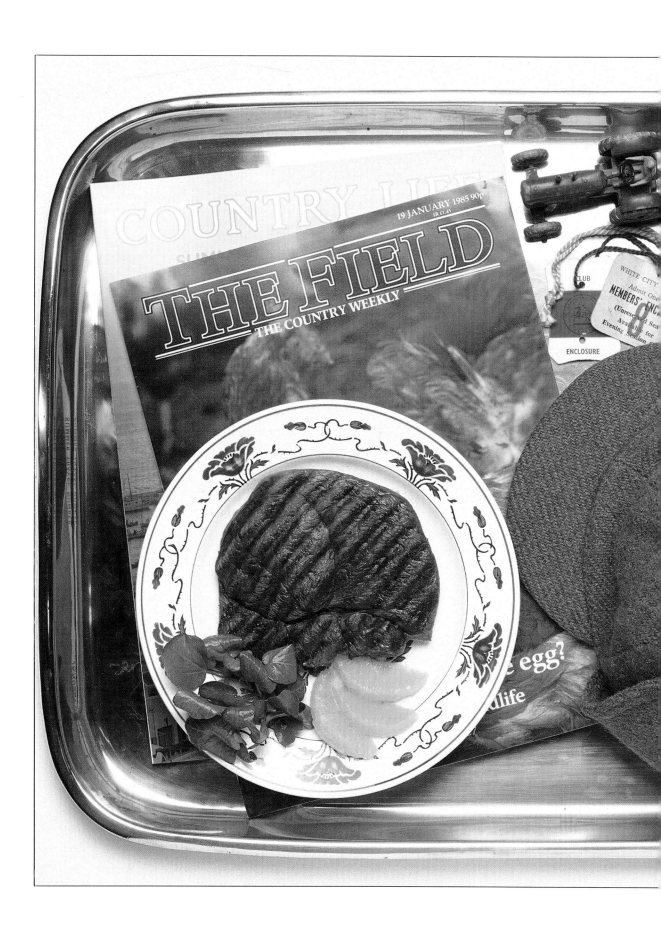

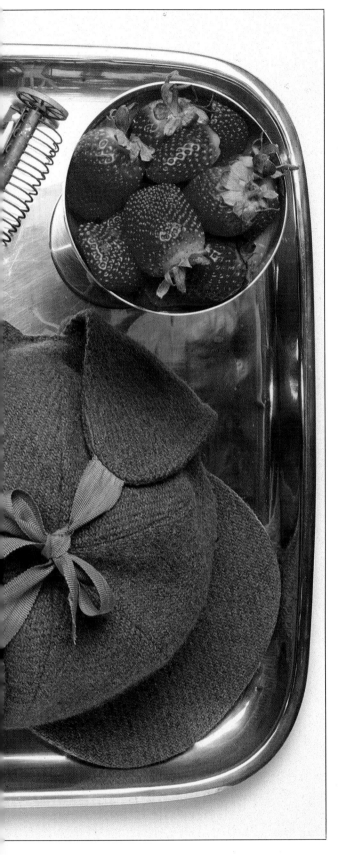

LANDED GENTRY DAY

Today you can wear off a few extra calories by nodding sagely as you listen to the manager's reports on the state of your nation.

BREAKFAST

Poached haddock
Poached egg
Unsweetened black tea or coffee

Poached haddock

Do not buy boil-in-the-bag or those luridly coloured 'golden cutlets'. Smoked haddock should have a delicate, very pale, gold-creamy colour. If it doesn't, go to another fishmonger. To poach the fish, put the fillets into a shallow frying pan and pour the milk over them. Simmer on top of the cooker; it should take about 10 minutes. For inexplicable reasons smoked haddock always takes longer to cook than it ought to, so after the first 10 minutes check to see that it's flaky and tender – if not, keep going.

You may eat the poached haddock as it is with just lemon juice and pepper, but for a more substantial breakfast you can top it with a poached egg. To poach eggs bring to the boil some salted water to which a *very* small amount of vinegar has been added. Break the egg into a teacup and then slide it from the teacup into the boiling water. Use two spoons to keep the white from drifting away from the yolk. Cover and boil for about 4 minutes. There are egg poachers for the inept, but the results are never as good as with this 'free form' way.

LUNCH

Cold roast pheasant
Watercress and orange salad

Cold roast pheasant

1 pheasant
olive oil
1 onion
2 ribs celery, chopped
salt and pepper

Pheasant, our most popular and readily to hand game, too often sounds much better than it tastes. Its often elusive merits require most ginger treatment – a badly cooked pheasant is a dry and miserable tasting thing. One should also dispatch the elaborate mythology about 'highness' and excessive hanging of the birds. You should not hang them until they are rotten and falling to bits – anyone should have the sense to stop short of total putrification. A young bird needn't be hung for more than four days. An old bird can be hung and hung and still never be good enough for plain roasting – it will have to be cooked in a high calorie casserole. The French, perverse in so many things, like their pheasant underdone – not such a bad idea as the birds pass the critical stage quite quickly. You will, of course, either shoot the pheasant yourself or be given it by shooting friends. *Buying* the bird smacks of *arrivisme*.

Manly sportsmen may baulk at watercress and orange salad, with its overtones of fey nouvellesque cookery, but press on bravely – the silly idea of fruit with one's main course really works in this case.

Cold roast pheasant is particularly good, and if you take the time to prepare this in advance, you will have a lunch fit for a mega landlord. The most sensible low-fat way of cooking the bird is in a chicken brick, which eliminates the need for barding with bacon fat.

Rub the pheasant lightly with olive oil. Place a peeled and quartered onion and some celery in the body cavity. Season with salt and pepper. Put the pheasant into the brick. Put the brick in a cold oven, turn on to 450°F/230°C/Gas mark 8 and leave for about 1½ hours for the average cock pheasant. Smaller hens will take a bit less time. Have a look at your pheasant after an hour – it's ready when the juices run clear after the thickest part of the leg has been pricked with a fork.

The thinly sliced half breast of a pheasant should be more than enough for lunch. Remember to remove the skin.

Sliced cold pheasant is wonderfully well accompanied by a salad of watercress and orange. Take as much watercress as you like (being almost calorie free, it doesn't matter), wash well in cold water, dry and put into a bowl with an orange cut up into segments. Toss very lightly with oil, vinegar, salt and pepper.

DINNER

The increasing availability of reared game may cheer the anti-blood-sport lobby, but salmon, partridge and pheasant all have to be wild to be good. Venison is the great exception, indeed, I slightly prefer the taste of farmed venison and applaud the ease with which I can now buy it. Lean and flavourful, it is remarkably good for the dieter as long as venison stews and roasts with heavy sauces are shunned.

Grilled venison steaks

2 7oz/200g venison steaks

Heat your grill very hot. I like to use the cast-iron grill that sits on top of the burner on a cooker, but any grill will really do. Lightly oil either side of the venison. These steaks should be cooked rare. Grill for about 5 minutes, then turn and grill the other side for a further 5 minutes. These times are obviously approximate: grilling times vary tremendously with the heat of the grill and the thickness of the meat. When cooked, slice thinly and spice liberally with fresh black pepper.

They are also excellent with Francatelli's venison sauce, as recorded by Jane Grigson in *Good Things*: Simmer together for 5 minutes 2 tablespoons port, ½ tablespoon redcurrant jelly, a small cinammon stick and a little grated lemon rind.

Puréed celeriac

1 knob celeriac
lemon juice
butter
salt and pepper

Celeriac, a most underrated and unfairly scorned vegetable, is especially good with venison. Wash the dirt from a knob of celeriac in cold water and then peel the ugly looking root – this is tiresome, but not frightfully difficult. Slice and put the slices in cold water with a few drops of lemon juice to keep from discolouring. Boil in salted water for 20 to 25 minutes, until quite soft, then purée in a mouli or food processor. Add just a tiny walnut-sized bit of butter, salt and pepper.

Venison and celeriac are both quite substantial so you should only have either a very light salad – maybe cos lettuce and chervil – or some fresh fruit afterwards.

A fairly tough Burgundy or one of the heavier Beaujolais, like a Morgon, is quite good with this.

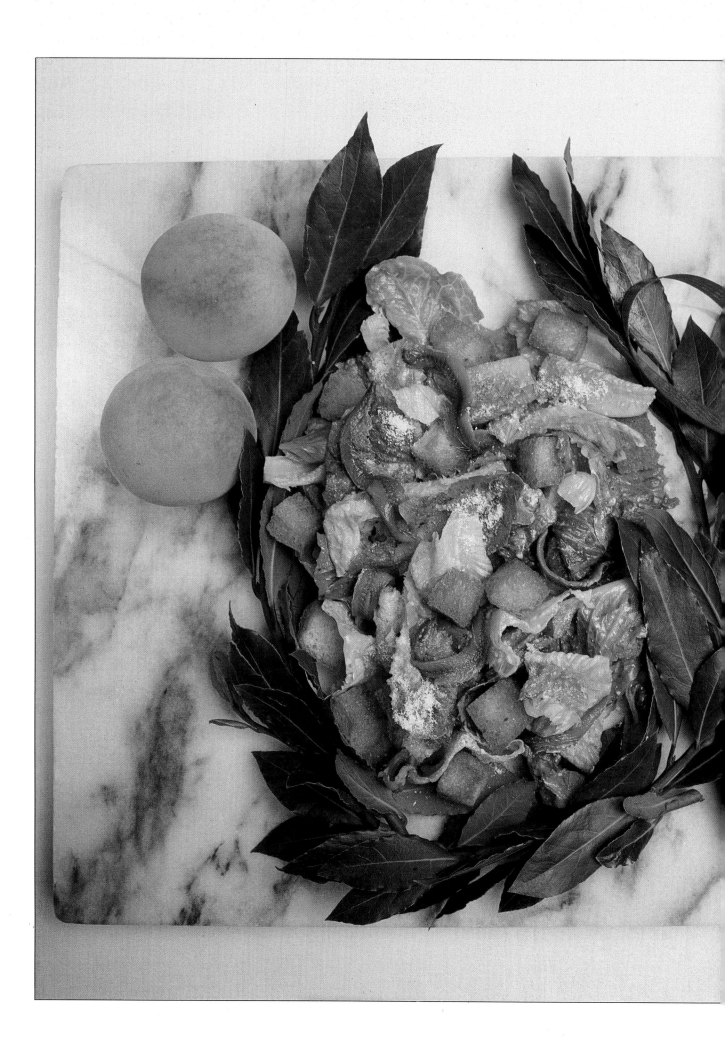

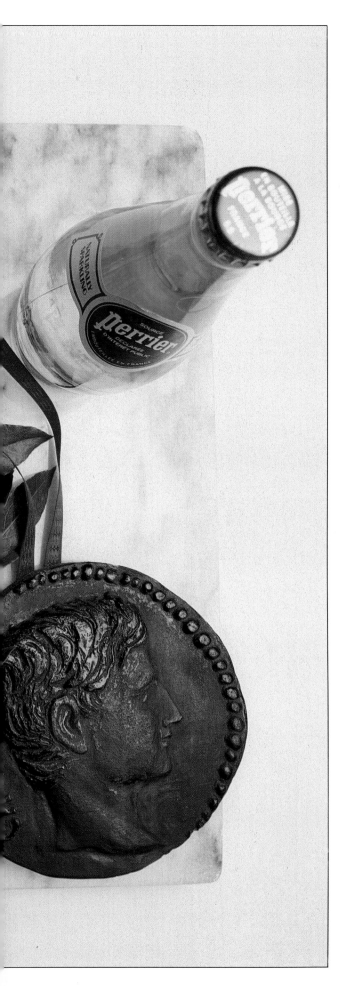

ROMAN EMPEROR'S DAY

The banquets of Imperial Rome are the exemplar of depraved gourmandism. Anyone who wishes to practise the Roman custom of self-induced vomiting may consume unlimited quantities of larks' tongues, bear paws and hummingbird wings. The less coarse may wish to accompany today's recipes with readings from Suetonius.

BREAKFAST

> *1 whole grapefruit*
> *Unsweetened black coffee or tea*

You are now entering the stage where grapefruit boredom becomes a major hazard to mental stability. Fortunately, it's not hard to overcome. Remember that early in the morning you're not sufficiently *compos mentis* to know what you're eating. And ease the pain by choosing grapefruits carefully – some of the brutes can be too much of a short sharp shock in the morning. Buy pink grapefruits if you can: that's what they eat in Dallas and look how rich those cowboys are. *In extremis* you may spike your grapefruit with a shot of ice cold vodka – if so, work from home that day.

LUNCH

> *Tomato and onion salad*
> *Grilled fillet steak*
> *French beans*
> *Mineral water*
> *Unsweetened black coffee or tea*

The salad should be well-seasoned with basil and black pepper, the steak eaten rare, and the beans garnished with lemon juice. One ought to drink Italian mineral water. The slightly obscure Fiuggi – still and rather alkaline – much loved by Michelangelo, will keep you on your toes. If lunching alone, Italian mineral waters are invariably best – all those endorsements by obscure pro-hydro-therapy dons make for enthralling reading.

DINNER

Caesar Salad is, appropriately, the most majestic dish in the salad world. Like the Niçoise, it is problematical in both ingredients and method of preparation. The admirable and adventurous Julia Child tracked down the daughter of the salad's creator, Tijuana restaurateur Caesar Cardini (you really thought this was a relic of Julius's time?!), and printed the definitive recipe in her book *From Julia Child's Kitchen*. I find her version delicious, but really not quite right, so here is the one I prefer.

Caesar Salad

4 large cloves garlic
4 tbsp finest olive oil
1 cos lettuce
2 eggs
2 tbsp freshly grated Parmesan cheese
5 anchovy fillets, finely chopped
croûtons

Peel and chop or crush the garlic. Add it to the olive oil. Discard the unattractive outer leaves of the lettuce, rinse remaining leaves thoroughly and dry in a salad spinner. Tear into bite-size pieces and put into a huge bowl. Pour the oil and garlic mixture over the lettuce and toss thoroughly so that the leaves are evenly covered in the oil. Put the eggs into boiling water for 1 minute only. (This sounds like very little time but any longer and the eggs will overcook.) Crack the eggs and add the yolks to the salad bowl. Toss thoroughly again to distribute the yolks. Add the Parmesan cheese and anchovy fillets. Toss again and finally add a generous sprinkling of home-made or commercially prepared croûtons.

It is vital to note that you cannot use any lettuce other than cos (round lettuce tastes of nothing and iceberg can't be properly coated with this dressing) and that the Parmesan must not be that stuff that comes out of a packet and gives everything the taste of last night's take-away pizza. As you refine your Caesar making ability, you'll be able to judge the proper seasoning by smell – the scents of the garlic and Parmesan should be pretty evenly balanced. If you can't bear anchovies (and it seems a surprising number of people can't), you may instead add three or four drops of Worcestershire sauce: our modern equivalent of the garum with which Romans dosed all their cookery.

As this salad is strongly flavoured, but doesn't contain any vinegar, you can amuse yourself by trying to find a decent white wine that is assertive enough to stand up to the onslaught of so much garlic and anchovies. A really good Italian white like a Greco di Tufo or a Gavi goes well with this.

Nothing else is needed to accompany this salad, and a fairly sweet fruit, such as a very ripe peach, would make a good dessert.

DAY 7

SCOTTISH LAIRD'S DAY

Halfway, halfway. As the pounds slip away, your increased agility at strip the willow will no doubt pay social dividends next St Andrew's Day.

As a lifelong devotee of porridge, I regret its omission. While recent evidence shows that the soluble fibre contained in oats is excellent for slimmers, it is sad to relate that porridge (whether eaten up standing up or sitting down – a debate that carries on) cannot be consumed without enormous quantities of brown sugar or golden syrup or both so you will have to wait until next winter.

BREAKFAST

½ grapefruit
Jugged kippers
Unsweetened black tea or coffee

Jugged kippers

There are kippers and kippers: fearsome kippers that come in plastic bags and sublime kippers that come from the Isle of Man or the Yorkshire coast or Loch Fyne or Craster. Don't compromise on your kipper. Most people find the smell of breakfast-time grilled kippers overpowering (especially in the evening – the smell is remarkably tenacious). Jugged kippers are less pungent and just as delicious. Put kippers (one per person) head down in a jug and pour boiling water straight from the kettle over them. Leave for 10 minutes, drain and there you have it.

LUNCH

Poached salmon
Petits pois
Green salad
Highland Spring mineral water
Unsweetened black tea or coffee

DINNER

Roast partridge with wild rice
Endive salad
Baked bananas en papillote

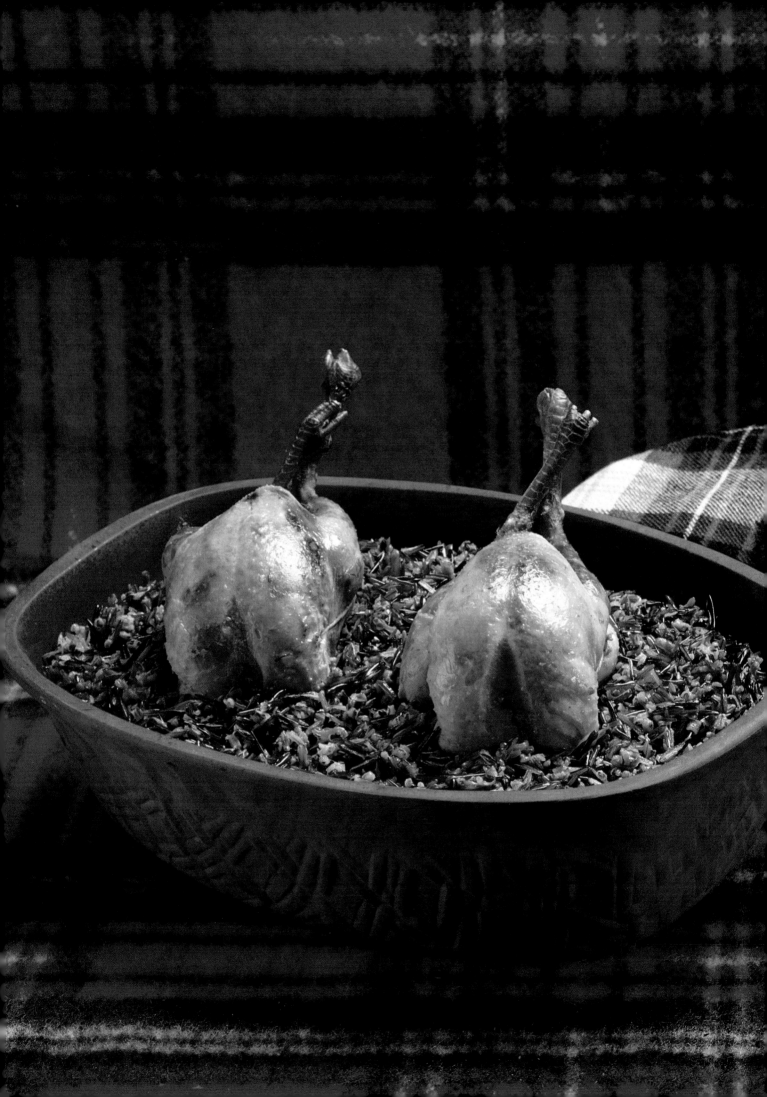

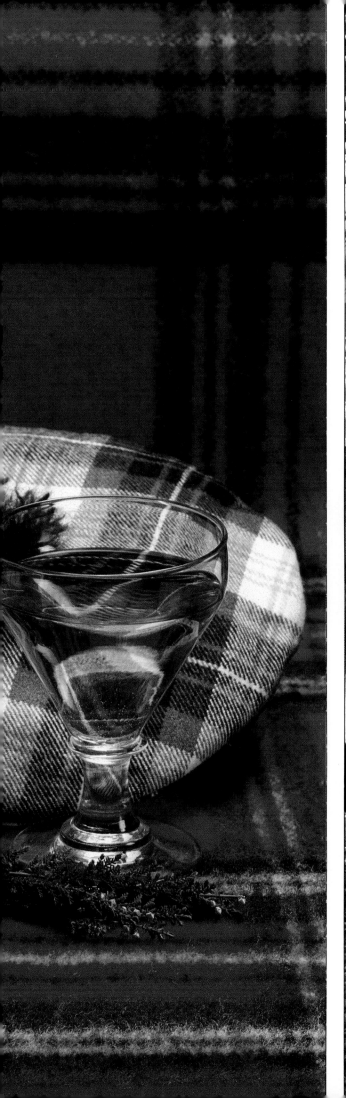

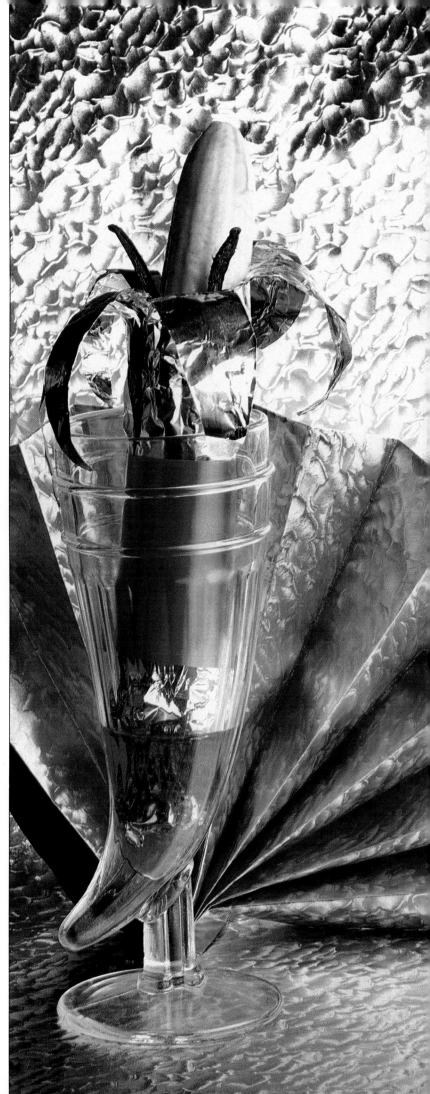

Partridge is the best of all game birds. Alas, its fondness for arable land combined with our farmers' overuse of dangerous pesticides means that the partridge population is declining. The Grey-legged Partridge is the most succulent, but even the Red-legged or French Partridge makes excellent eating. The partridge ought to be young; old birds get very tough and are good only for casseroles. Partridge, like any good specimen of bird, is at its best when simply roasted, but game birds tend to be dry and have to be barded with extraneous fat to keep them moist when cooking. This barding, with its unwelcome calories, can be dispensed with if you cook the birds in a chicken brick.

Roast partridge

Take two young partridges, brush them with olive oil and place them breast up in the bottom of a chicken brick. Surround them with quartered onions or a liberal sprinkling of chopped shallots. Cover the brick and place it in a cold oven. Then set the oven very hot – 450°F/230°C/Gas mark 8. After about 1 hour the birds will be done. I usually leave them in a bit longer, as I like my partridge be thoroughly cooked with just the barest tinge of pink. However, do be especially wary of overcooking.

Wild Rice

Wild rice is marvellously good with roast birds, but, like partridge, is becoming an endangered species to anyone except a millionaire because of its very high price. A good alternative if one's capital is otherwise engaged is one of the superior grades of Italian brown rice.

1½oz/40g butter
2 tbsp chopped shallots
8oz/225g wild rice
8fl oz/240ml chicken stock or water

Melt the butter in the bottom of a saucepan and cook the chopped shallots until they become translucent. Pour in the wild rice and fry gently until the grains are well coated with the butter. Add the chicken stock or water and boil for 2 minutes. Reduce the heat, cover and simmer gently and undisturbed for about 25 minutes. Inspect the rice and you should find tender grains and a series of little holes on the surface. If these signs haven't appeared, replace the lid and continue cooking until they do.

Follow with a salad of endive dressed in a very light olive oil.

Baked bananas en papillote

It has been said that no gentleman eats cooked bananas, but this prejudice is disappearing. This simple and very tasty pudding is derived from Michel Guerard's *Cuisine Minceur* recipe.

2 ripe bananas
1 vanilla pod
2 tbsp dark rum

Peel and place each banana in the centre of a rectangle of aluminium foil. Split open the vanila pod and place one half next to each banana. Pour 1 tablespoon of rum over each banana. Fold the aluminium foil and crimp the edges tightly to make two packages. Bake at 425°F/220°C/Gas mark 7 for about 20 minutes. Eat while still very hot.

A perfect roast partridge deserves your finest half-bottle of claret – go on, bring the Pétrus up from the cellar.

DAY 8

BILLIONAIRE'S DAY

Abandoning the flashy vulgarity of common or garden millionairism, today's diet aims at more discreet consumption. When you have this much money, you don't have to flaunt it.

BREAKFAST

1 glass fresh orange juice
Billionaire's Bran Flakes
Lapsang Souchong tea

Billionaire's bran flakes

1 tbsp chopped dates
1 tbsp chopped hazlenuts
4 oz/100g bran flakes
Skimmed milk

Place all the ingredients together in a small bowl, and consider as you enter the second half of this dietary regime that your fortune is flourishing while your girth is diminishing.

LUNCH

Consommé
Grilled lamb chops
Mixed salad
Mineral water
Unsweetened black tea or coffee

Canned beef consommé is an indispensable item for quick snacks. Chilled and slightly tarted up, it makes a good first course. Chill a 15 fl oz/450 ml can of consommé in the refrigerator for at least 2 hours. Open the can, break up the jellied consommé with a fork and divide it into two well-chilled two-handled cups. Top each helping with 1 tablespoon of sour cream and about 1 oz/25 g of decent Sevruga caviar.

Lamb chops tend to be fatty, so they are best grilled on a conventional grilling tray with a drip pan underneath rather than directly on a hot cast-iron grill. You must also exercise the considerable restraint needed to avoid eating the delicious but forbidden charred lamb fat.

A mixed salad of sliced tomato, a thinly sliced carrot, a few well-chopped spring onions and some Webb lettuce goes well. If salad boredom sets in, you can always jazz up salads by the addition of cold cooked kidney or cannellini beans, or some chickpeas.

DINNER

> *Salmon and sorrel* en papillote
> *Strawberry and kiwi fruit salad*

One of the nicest ways to cook fish is *en papil-lote*, sealed up in an envelope, so that it cooks in its own juices (with a little outside help). Let each person open his own envelope – the aroma is sensational.

Salmon and sorrel en papillote

8oz/225g sorrel
1oz/25g butter
2 salmon steaks
salt and pepper
dash of white wine

Sorrel, a relation of the dock weed we have all used to sooth nettle stings, is excellent with any rich fish, particularly salmon. Chop the sorrel and cook for just a few minutes in melted butter to soften and make it slightly less sour. Take two large rectangles of aluminium foil and put half the cooked sorrel in the centre of each one. Place a salmon steak on top, season with salt and pepper and add a dash of white wine for extra moisture. Then fold over the edges of the rec-tangle to make a well-sealed little parcel – neat-ness does *not* count. Put the parcels onto a baking tray and cook in a medium oven 350°F/180°C/Gas mark 4 for 20–25 minutes. Always make a surreptitious check before serving, as undercooked salmon is not at all nice. This salmon doesn't really need another vegetable with it.

Strawberry and kiwi fruit salad

Slice as many strawberries as you like. Add a sliced kiwi fruit and top each portion with one tablespoon of Grand Marnier – and, yes, *one* tablespoon is enough.

You can enjoy this meal with as good a white burgundy as you can afford – and money is no object to you, is it? – or with one of those great California chardonnays.

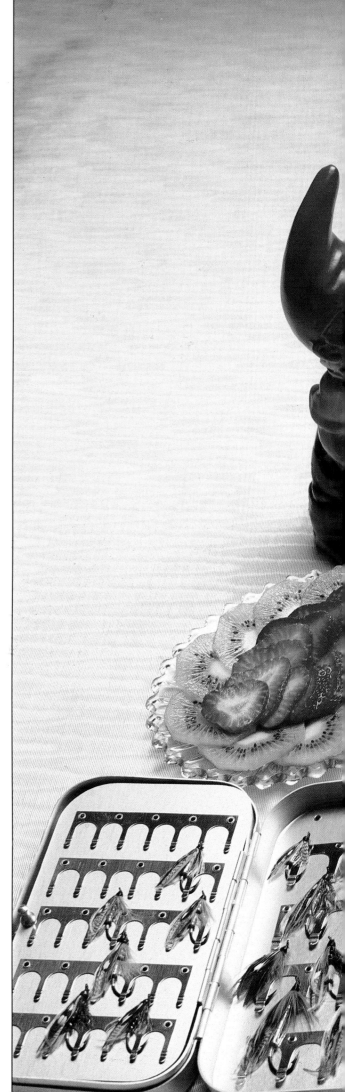

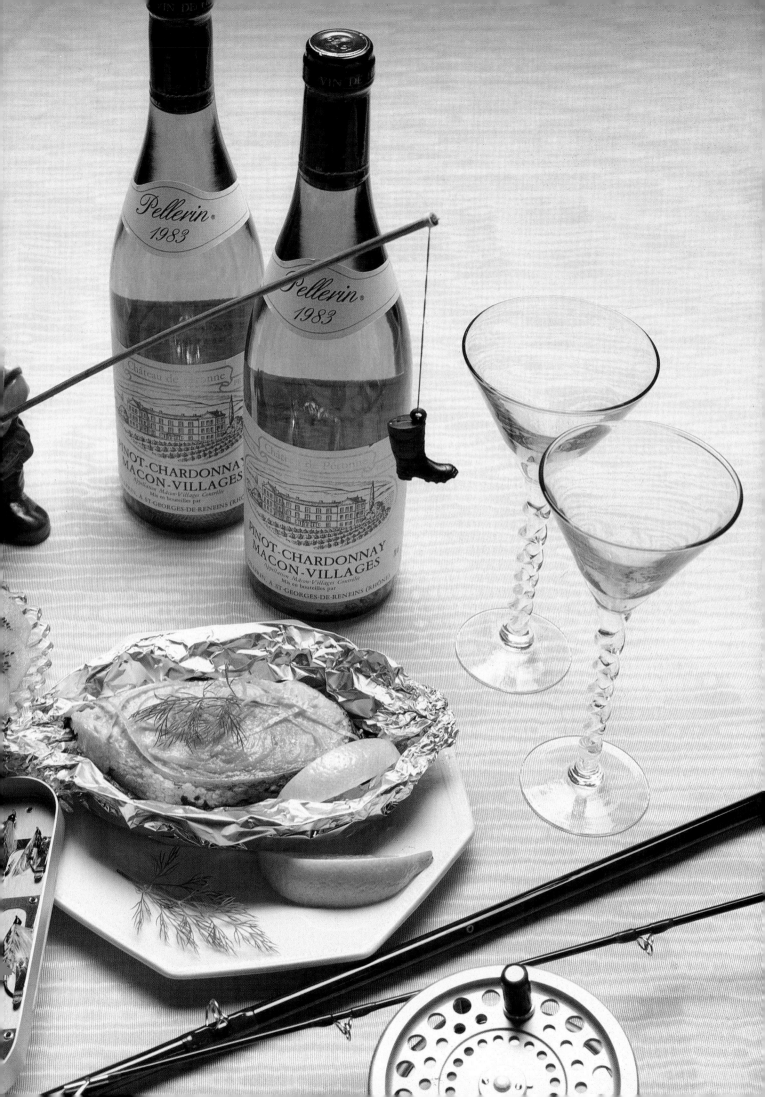

DAY 9

BELGIAN BANKER'S DAY

Some rich people are boring and no amount of effort will make them interesting. Bankerly conservatism, while economically laudable, has no place at the dinner table.

BREAKFAST

Glass fresh orange juice
½ pot yoghurt
1 banana
Unsweetened black tea or coffee

You must by now become more adventurous with your tea drinking, as unblinded by milk and sugar you will be able to appreciate the subtle flavours. Green tea is far too insipid for breakfast, but you should get a kick out of a really first rate oolong or a Russian Caravan tea.

LUNCH

White asparagus
Grilled turbot
Endive salad

When Ludwig Bemelmans – the only first-rate waiter who was also a first-rate writer – returned to Munich after the Great War he entertained his former tutor, Professor Hellsgang, to lunch. As a first course Bemelmans, who was by then a big shot in the New York hotel trade, ordered half a dozen white asparagus each. The Professor ate his first three asparagus with ecstasy and then took out his pocket handkerchief, wrapped up the remaining three and slipped them into his coat pocket. 'For my wife' he explained. 'We haven't seen asparagus since before the war.'

Emulate Bemelmans and make this a lunch for two.

White asparagus

Belgians, Germans and French are fond of white asparagus, which are harvested before the shoots have broken through the topsoil. The giant French *argenteuil* and the Belgian *malines* asparagus are, I think, far less tasty than the green English asparagus, but they make an amusing change and certainly add more Belgian flavour. Serve hot, cold or tepid, with either a tiny bit of hot or warm melted butter or cold vinaigrette and lots of black pepper. Do not ever buy those tins or bottles of white asparagus – they are hideously overpriced, and not at all nice to eat.

The unpleasant reaction between the sulphur in asparagus and wine is a further incentive to lay off the Burgundy at lunchtime; drink Spa instead.

44

Grilled turbot

Noble but with a dangerous tendency to extreme dullness, the turbot is unsurprisingly the favourite fish of the Belgians. When there's turbot on the table, you know a Belgian likes you. Indeed, during my first trip to Belgium there was turbot at five out of six meals. Classically (it was the favourite fish of the satirist Juvenal) the turbot is poached in a large diamond shaped vessel made for the purpose and known as a *turbotier*. A *turbotier* is not easy to find, but do not bother to send your staff in search of one; few households require a whole poached turbot, and as it must be swathed in hollandaise, which is anathema to any diet, you would do well to avoid it. The fish is much nicer grilled and dressed with a squeeze of fresh lemon juice and black pepper.

Smear 2 turbot steaks with a small amount of oil – just enough to barely coat them – and dust them lightly with flour. Be sure that the steaks aren't too thick – say, no more than 1½ inches/35 mm. Take a cast-iron fish grill or frying pan and heat it until very hot. Lower the heat to medium and put the steaks on the grill. It is difficult to lay down rules about cooking times, as there are far too many variables involved, but after about 5 minutes you should be able to turn the fish over. Continue cooking for another 5 minutes. Cooking directly on a hot iron grill will give you a crispy, slightly charred crust and succulent insides, although constant vigilance and practice are required.

This turbot is best followed by a salad on the Belgian theme – some sliced endive dressed with a little walnut oil and red wine vinegar.

There is no Belgian wine and sadly their most excellent beer doesn't really go well with turbot. This upmarket fish deserves a good half bottle of an important white burgundy – don't be mean with the Montrachet and remember this is your only chance to drink half bottles.

DINNER
Smoked turkey and mango with salad

8oz/225g sliced smoked turkey
1 very ripe mango
lettuce
radicchio
spring onions
walnut oil

Really good smoked turkey is excellent for diets, as it is terribly lean and the thin layer of fatty skin on top of each slice peels off easily. Have your butcher or delicatessen slice it quite thickly – as you would with roast turkey – rather than into the customary paper-thin slices, which really are awfully prissy. Turkey does tend to be dry, and while the traditional accompaniments of brandied peaches and mayonnaise are, unfortunately, off-limits, the more exotic mango will provide consolation.

Take the very ripe mango and julienne it finely. Make a mound of it in the centre of a serving plate and arrange the sliced smoked turkey around it. The succulence and slight tang of the mango are a perfect counterpart to the vaguely austere turkey.

Serve a simple mixed salad with this: mâche (or if mâche is not available, cos lettuce), radicchio and finely chopped spring onions taste very good dressed in a little walnut oil.

Gewürztraminer is a delightful accompaniment to this salad.

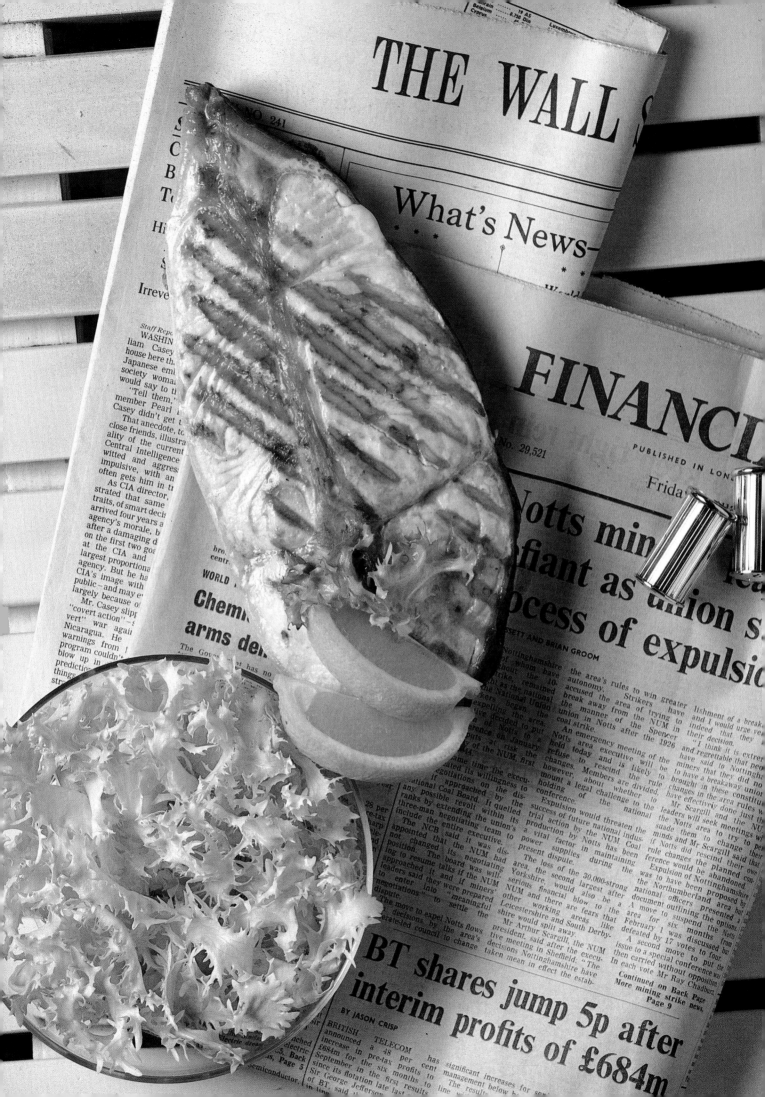

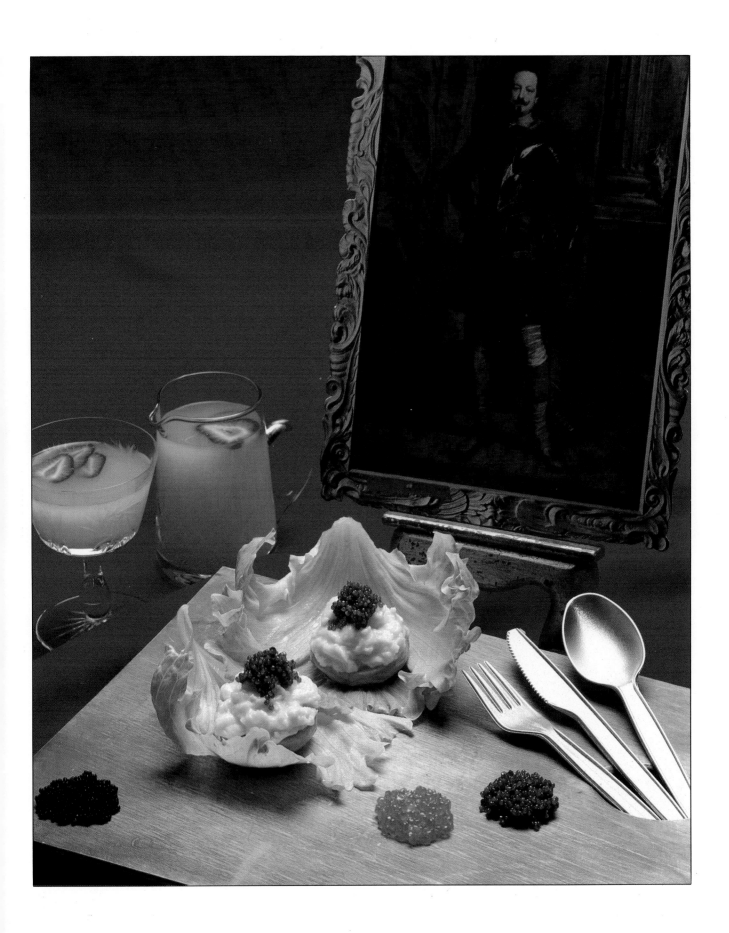

DAY 10

MULTIMILLIONAIRE'S DAY

No number of off-shore corporations, tax shelters or 'registered charities' will let you take it with you, so spread some of the wealth around your local food shops.

BREAKFAST

Fresh grapefruit juice
Scrambled Eggs Van Dyck
Unsweetened black tea or coffee

This breakfast is so wonderful that it's worth sharing: make it for two.

Scrambled Eggs Van Dyck

2 artichokes
2 tbsp flour
3½ pt/2 l water
juice of 1 lemon
4 eggs
black pepper
1 oz/25 g unsalted butter
4 oz/100 g Sevruga caviar

Preparing artichoke bottoms is rather time-consuming, but not as frightful as it sounds. I like this method used by Louisette Bertholle in *French Cooking for All*.

Twist the stems off the artichokes. Snap off all the outside leaves, but don't touch the tender bunch of whitish leaves in the centre of the artichoke. In a small mixing bowl add enough water to the flour to make the consistency of double cream and stir this mixture into a large saucepan containing the 3½ pt/2 l of water. Add the juice of a lemon and bring to the boil. Put in the artichokes and boil for about 20 minutes; old or large artichokes may take longer. They are ready when you can easily pierce the bottom with a knife. Drain them upside down in a colander, remove the leaves and hairy choke and put them aside in a covered dish to keep warm.

Break the eggs into a mixing bowl and beat them with some fresh black pepper. Melt the butter in a saucepan, pour in the beaten eggs and stir vigilantly over a low heat until the eggs become quite creamy. Place a heap of the scrambled eggs over each artichoke bottom and top each helping with half the caviar (no point in being *too* extravagant).

Remind yourself this is a diet by consuming a cup of unsweetened black tea or coffee.

LUNCH

12 oysters
Blackberries and sliced peach
Unsweetened black tea or coffee

You may be allergic to oysters; if so, you know by now – otherwise the fear of bad oysters is irrational. Oysters from a reputable oyster man or from a first class restaurant are rarely 'bad'. Lemon juice and black pepper are the only seasonings needed. Vinegar on oysters is not a mistake, but a tragedy.

DINNER

Turtle soup
Cold boiled lobster
Green salad

Turtle soup

1 15 fl oz/450 ml can turtle soup
1 tbsp Madeira
squeeze of lemon juice

The Madeira and lemon juice will enliven the canned soup, which, served will whet your appetite (surely by this point in the regime your appetite is diminishing) for the lobster.

Cold boiled lobster

Lobster is unquestionably the best thing to come out of the sea. The larger North American lobster (*Homarus americanus*) is slightly tastier than its close European relation (*Homarus gammarus*), but both Atlantic lobsters are far superior to the clawless spiny lobsters. Probably the two best ways to eat lobster are stuffed with savoury breadcrumbs and baked (as is most commonly found in New England) or hot boiled. Unfortunately, both must be served with staggering quantities of melted butter – more than enough to destroy any dietary regime. The next best thing – and it really is no hardship – is cold boiled lobster, which need be served only with generous amounts of lemon and black pepper. You may wish to boil the unfortunate crustacean yourself, in which case you merely plunge it into some vigorously boiling water and wait 15 minutes for a chicken lobster (one that weighs just over 1 lb/450 g but under 1½ lb/675 g). If you have a good reliable fishmonger, as you ought to, you may buy a boiled lobster from him.

Serve the lobster with a straightforward green salad of, perhaps, cos lettuce and a healthy handful of chopped chives.

If you wish to drink champagne, be sure that it is an extremely dry one, like Bollinger – no airline champagne allowed with this meal. If bored with Bollinger, you would do just as well to drink a great white burgundy.

Unsweetened tea or coffee is the regrettable anti-climax to this day.

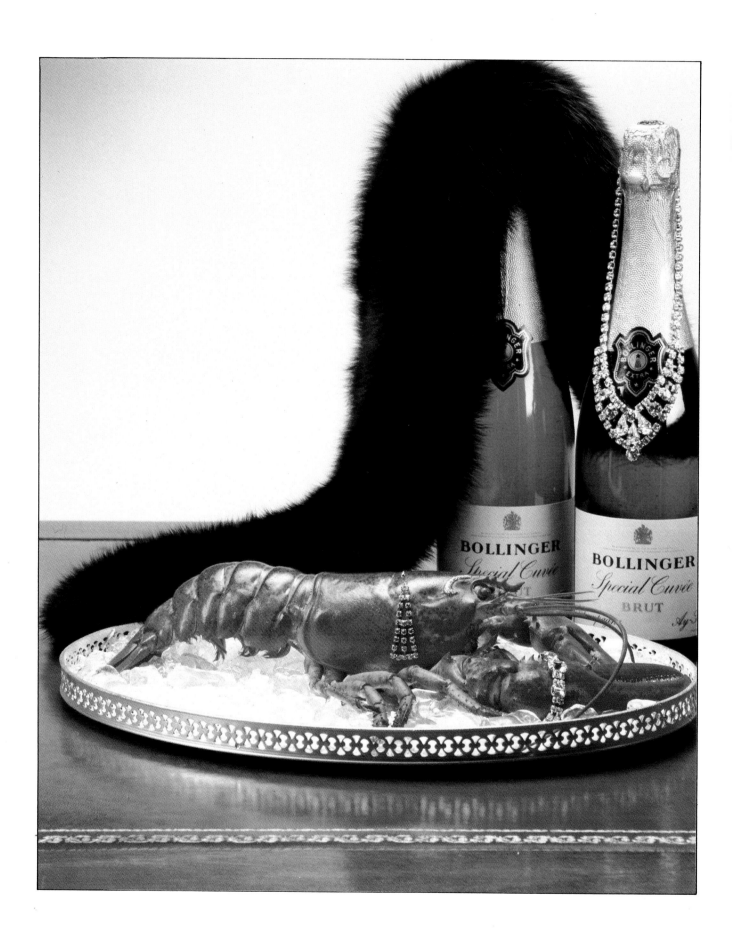

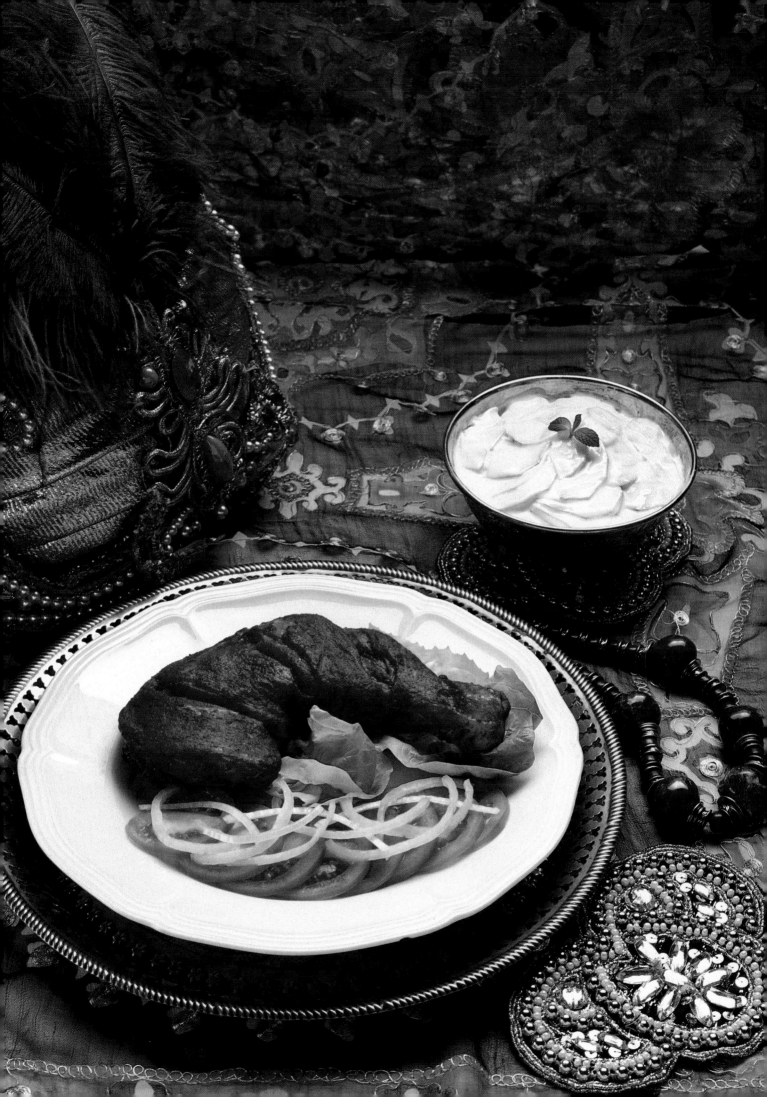

MULTINATIONAL MOGUL'S DAY

BREAKFAST

Fresh grapefruit juice
Sliced pawpaw
Unsweetened black coffee or tea

LUNCH

Tandoori chicken
Mixed salad
Raita

Tandoori chicken

2 chicken breasts with skin
lemon juice
salt
4 cloves garlic
2 tsp ground ginger
1 tsp pickling spice
1/2 tsp ground cumin
1/2 tbsp white wine vinegar
5 oz/150g yoghurt
2 tsp paprika
butter

Tandoori chicken ought to be cooked in a tandoor Indian clay oven, of course, but few of us have one at home and domestic versions on the market aren't entirely satisfactory. The tirelessly inventive Josceline Dimbleby has concocted a perfectly good home version, which I've adapted.

Make deep cuts in the chicken breasts and rub with lemon juice and salt. Allow to sit for about 30 minutes. Blend the garlic, ground ginger, pickling spice, ground cumin, white wine vinegar, yoghurt, and paprika in a liquidizer and smear over the chicken breasts. Leave overnight in the fridge. Heat your oven to 400°F/200°C/Gas mark 6, place the chicken in a roasting pan, dot with butter and cook for 20 minutes. Sprinkle with lemon juice, baste with melted butter and grill each side under a hot grill for about 5 minutes.

You will want to serve this with a simple mixed salad or maybe a tomato and onion salad dressed with a tiny bit of oil.

Raita is a nicely cooling accompaniment. Merely add half a finely sliced cucumber and five well chopped dates to a small bowl of yoghurt.

DINNER

Asparagus risotto
Green salad
Unsweetened black tea or coffee

A real risotto is an immensely luxurious dish miles far removed from the greasy mixtures of overcooked rice and left-overs so often served.

Asparagus risotto

With the development of commercial market gardening and the transport of food by railway, asparagus almost went out of fashion. In Zola's *Paris* the rich and villainous Baron Duvillard reluctantly offers his luncheon guests some asparagus *a primeur*, which once had been so rare, but which no longer caused any astonishment. 'Nowadays we get it all the winter' said the Baron with a gesture of disenchantment. The cricket-bat-size giants from California and Spain are okay, but lack that springtime brilliance of the first English asparagus.

Arborio rice has stubby grains and makes a creamy risotto. If you can't find arborio, you may substitute American long grain, but the result won't be quite the same.

6 oz/175 g arborio rice
½ lb/450 g fresh asparagus
½ onion, sliced
12 fl oz/350 ml chicken stock
1½ oz/40 g butter
1 tbsp Parmesan cheese
salt and pepper

Prepare the asparagus by peeling them with a swivel peeler beginning about 1½ inches/35 mm below the tip and peeling deeper as you approach the butt. This peeling seems finicky but makes for the best and most easily cooked asparagus. Throw the peeled asparagus into liberally-salted, ferociously boiling water and cook for 5 to 10 minutes. Do not overboil them — they are meant to look firm *not* impotent. Take about 12 fl oz/350 ml of the water you've boiled the asparagus in and mix it with an equal quantity of stock.

Melt the butter in the bottom of a heavy saucepan, and over fairly high heat sauté the sliced onions until translucent. Then cut the asparagus into 2-inch/50-mm pieces, add them to the pan and sauté them for just a few minutes. Add the rice and stir well; it will become shiny and well coated with the butter. Pour in 5-7 fl oz/150–200 ml of the stock mixture and stir the rice frequently. Add more of this liquid as the rice absorbs it. After about 25 minutes, begin tasting the rice. It should be well-cooked and unstarchy, but quite firm to the bite. When the rice is cooked — it will be surprisingly creamy — take it off the heat and let it rest for about 1 minute. Then add the freshly grated parmesan, salt and pepper as needed, and mix thoroughly.

The only accompaniment to this rather solid dish should be a well chosen green salad — cos and lambs lettuce, cress and some freshly chopped chervil.

Wine and asparagus are legendary enemies. You might serve a cheap Italian white with this, but would be far better off sticking to an Italian water like Madonna.

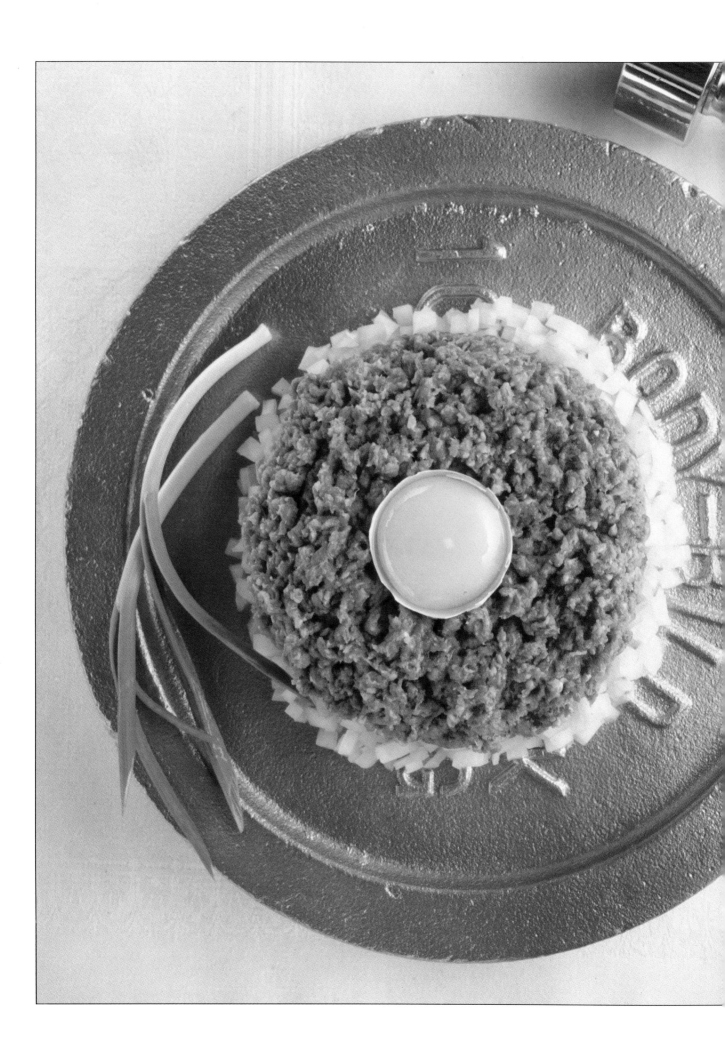

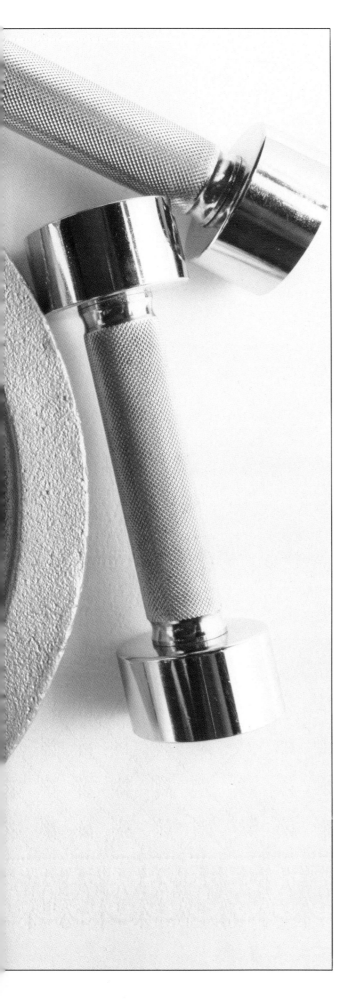

MILLIONAIRE'S MACHO DAY

Lévi-Strauss in his famous essay on steak and chips wrote how consuming beef had an almost magical aspect, giving the consumer a bull-like strength. The raw beef at the end of this day should make you even more bullish than usual.

BREAKFAST

> *Glass of fresh orange juice*
> *Cottage cheese*
> *Pear*
> *Unsweetened black tea or coffee*

LUNCH

> *Fetucelle with truffles*
> *Mâche and chervil salad*

Truffles have probably the strongest mystique of any luxury food. I suspect this may be because no one really likes them or indeed knows what to do with them. Too often they appear as a senseless and tasteless garnish. Their rarity and unequalled pungency have long made them a gourmet's favourite. Louis XVIII and his master of the household, the Duc d'Escars, were tireless gastronomes who enjoyed inventing recipes. One evening they concocted a new dish of ortolans (a once popular game bird now very rare) stuffed with a truffle purée: Escars died the next morning. Louis was unmoved by the courtier's demise: 'This only proves that what I've always said is true. I have the better stomach.'

Canned truffles are not particularly good, and of the two varieties of truffle on the market – black (perigord) truffles from France and white Italian truffles – I prefer the white. The smell can be off-putting to even the most dedicated fungiphile, being marginally more noisome than the reek of very dirty socks.

Cook 8 oz/225 g of fettucelle (see pasta cooking note, page 00) drain, divide onto two hot plates and add 1 tablespoon butter to each serving. Top with freshly sliced white truffle. Be very careful not to use too much truffle or an excess of pungency will render this most unpleasant.

Follow with a salad of mâche and chopped chervil tossed in a light vinaigrette.

DINNER

Ceviche
Steak Tartare
Green salad

Ceviche

Ceviche is not, strictly speaking, raw fish and so ought not to frighten even the most squeamish; it is simply fish that has been cooked without the agency of heat.

8 oz/225 g halibut, skinned and boned
or *scallops without the coral*
fresh lime or lemon juice
1 clove garlic, peeled
1 tbsp chopped onion
chopped chillies to taste

Cut the halibut into roughly 1-inch/25-mm cubes. (There are a number of variations. Instead of halibut you might use turbot, seabass or salmon – in which case dispense with the scallops.) Place in a small deep bowl and cover with fresh lemon or lime juice or a mixture of the two. You may find, as I do, that the scallops are better without their coral. Do not in any circumstances use frozen fish or frozen scallops for this dish – the result will be watery and revolting. Add the garlic, chopped onion and as many chopped chillies as you feel strong enough to handle. Don't be afraid of chillies; buy the most evil looking little brutes you can find – the shock is good for the system. Cover and keep in a cool place for 4-5 hours – you will notice that through the action of the citrus juice the fish has turned opaque like conventionally well-cooked fish. Some recipes call for a chopped coriander garnish, but I find that coriander's metallic taste doesn't do much for this dish. If you like a bit of green, you can garnish this with an ample amount of ordinary or flat-leafed (Italian) parsley. Serve with sliced tomatoes. This first course, like many others, also makes a good warm weather main course.

Steak Tartare

Like the Bloody Mary, its macho counterpart in the drinks world, Steak Tartare suffers much from the blood and guts pretentions of those who make it. The whole 'my steak tartare's more butch than yours' syndrome has got entirely out of hand. You must be firm but gentle, don't go overboard with Tabasco, mustard, capers or any of the other flavourings.

8oz/225g finest fillet steak (tell your butcher to
prepare it especially for steak tartare – you
cannot use even the best mince)

Season the steak with a bit of lemon juice, salt and pepper and divide it into two hamburger-shape patties. Press a half eggshell containing the yolk of an egg into the top centre of each patty and serve on a large chilled dish garnished with chopped onion, capers, anchovy fillets, and horseradish. Have bottles of Tabasco and Worcestershire sauce and a pot of Dijon mustard at the ready. The do-it-yourself non-cookery of Steak Tartare can be both amusing and rather educational. Mix your flavourings with restraint, though, or you could be staring at a fairly unpalatable mess.

As Steak Tartare is exceedingly rich, it is best served with a very simple green salad.

An assertive minor claret – some sort of Bergerac – goes well with this.

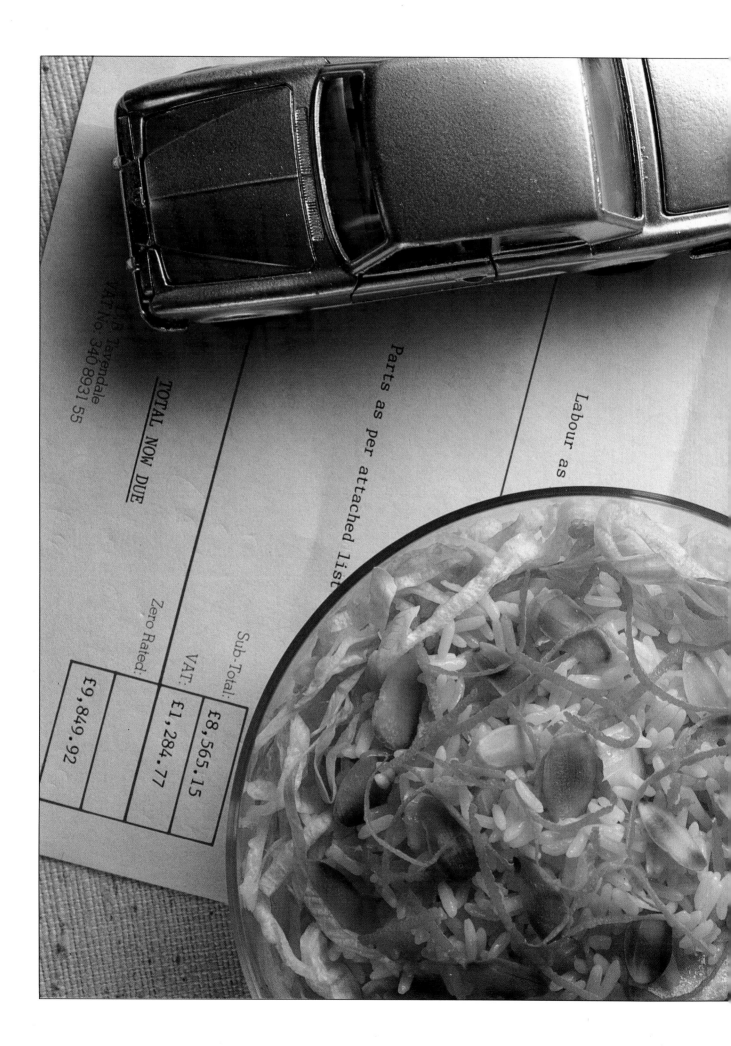

VAT No: 340 8931 55

TOTAL NOW DUE

Parts as per attached list

Labour as

Sub-Total: £8,565.15

VAT: £1,284.77

Zero Rated:

£9,849.92

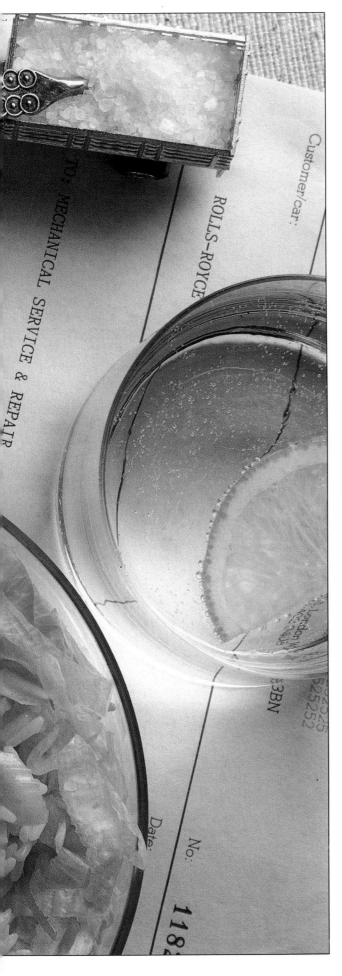

DAY 13

PAUPER'S DAY

The Roman Claudius Albinius is reputed (i.e. historians don't believe it, but it makes a nice story) to have dined on five hundred figs, a hundred peaches, ten melons and twenty pounds of grapes. This course of fruit is altogether less arduous.

BREAKFAST

> *Glass of fresh grapefruit juice infused with mint*
> *Half a Charente melon sliced and flavoured with 1 tbsp ginger wine*
> *Lapsang Souchong tea*

Fruit makes one feel awfully virtuous and close to the earth – do not let this unpleasant side effect deter you. If you can't find a nicely ripe Charente melon, any other sort will do with the egregious exception of watermelon – a fruit unfit for the table of the gentleborn although welcome at any picnic. Melons are also nice spiked with *eau de vie* – be sure to buy the proper ultraexpensive ones in glamorous bottles – or the current fashionable obsession of lemon-flavoured vodka. Do not exceed one tablespoon of any alcoholic embellishment – the flavour will be far too potent.

LUNCH

Cherry and Guava Salad

2 sliced guavas
4oz/100g cherries
2 tbsp red burgundy
1 tsp sugar

In a bowl combine the sliced guavas and the cherries. Moisten with the red burgundy to which the sugar has been added. If you don't like guavas, you may substitute some other tropical fruit like mango, for example. Keep a steady hand and a firm resolution when dealing with the sugar bowl. Wash down with unlimited sparkling water; the Swedish Ramlosa goes well with this.

DINNER

Orange Rice Salad

Robert Carrier's Orange Rice Salad (from his engaging *Quick Cook*) makes a good quasi-fruitarian main supper dish. You might think of it as a cold fruit rissotto.

2 tbsp finely chopped onion
1 stick finely chopped celery
olive oil
3 tbsp hot chicken stock
2 tbsp fresh orange juice
1 tbsp lemon juice
2 tsp grated orange rind
salt and pepper
4oz/100g cooked rice
toasted almonds
lettuce

Rice cookery is boring and problematical. The best method is as follows. Melt a little butter in a heavy saucepan. Add as much rice as needed and toss vigorously in the butter until the grains are translucent, then add a quantity of water equal to the volume of rice (say, one cup of rice needs one cup of water), salt and pepper, and bring to the boil for 3 minutes. Now reduce the heat, cover tightly, and go away. Twenty minutes later the rice will be cooked.

Sweat (i.e. soften without colouring) the onion and celery in a little olive oil for 5 minutes. Combine the hot chicken stock, fresh orange juice, lemon juice and grated orange rind. Season with salt and pepper. Put orange liquid, cooked vegetables and cooked rice in a saucepan and simmer for a few minutes until the liquid is absorbed. Chill, toss with a small amount of olive oil, scatter with toasted almonds and serve on a bed of lettuce.

For dessert serve 3 fresh figs per person dressed with ½ tablespoon of Pernod.

Enjoy with any fizzy water.

DAY 14

BIG SHOT'S DAY

Not quite so bloodthirsty as it sounds. Pheasant, of course, is still proper game (the excessively delicate can substitute guinea fowl) but farmed venison, of course, isn't.

BREAKFAST

Fresh orange juice
½ pot yoghurt
Papaya
Unsweetened black coffee or tea

Papayas are marvellously good to eat and do wonders for the digestion. They are most excellent puréed and used to flavour a very large glass of extremely dry champagne (have one tomorrow to celebrate your first day off the diet).

LUNCH

Cold pasta is frightfully good for the lunchbox, but needs to be prepared a day in advance.

4 oz/100 g fusilli, eliche or molle (all corkscrew shaped pastas)
3 large ripe tomatoes
1 clove garlic, peeled
1 tbsp best olive oil
5 drops Worcestershire sauce
1 tbsp freshly chopped basil
salt and pepper

Cook the pasta in plenty of well-salted boiling water until *al dente*, then drain and rinse thoroughly in cold water. Set aside to continue cooling. Peel, core and finely chop the tomatoes. Put them in a bowl with the garlic, olive oil, Worcestershire sauce and basil. Season with salt and pepper and let sit for at least 2 hours. Remove the clove of garlic and combine the sauce and pasta in a covered container and serve for lunch the next day (the longer they stay together the better).

Serve this with a very simple salad (hearts of iceberg lettuce dressed with lemon juice and black pepper), and an Italian water such as Crodo.

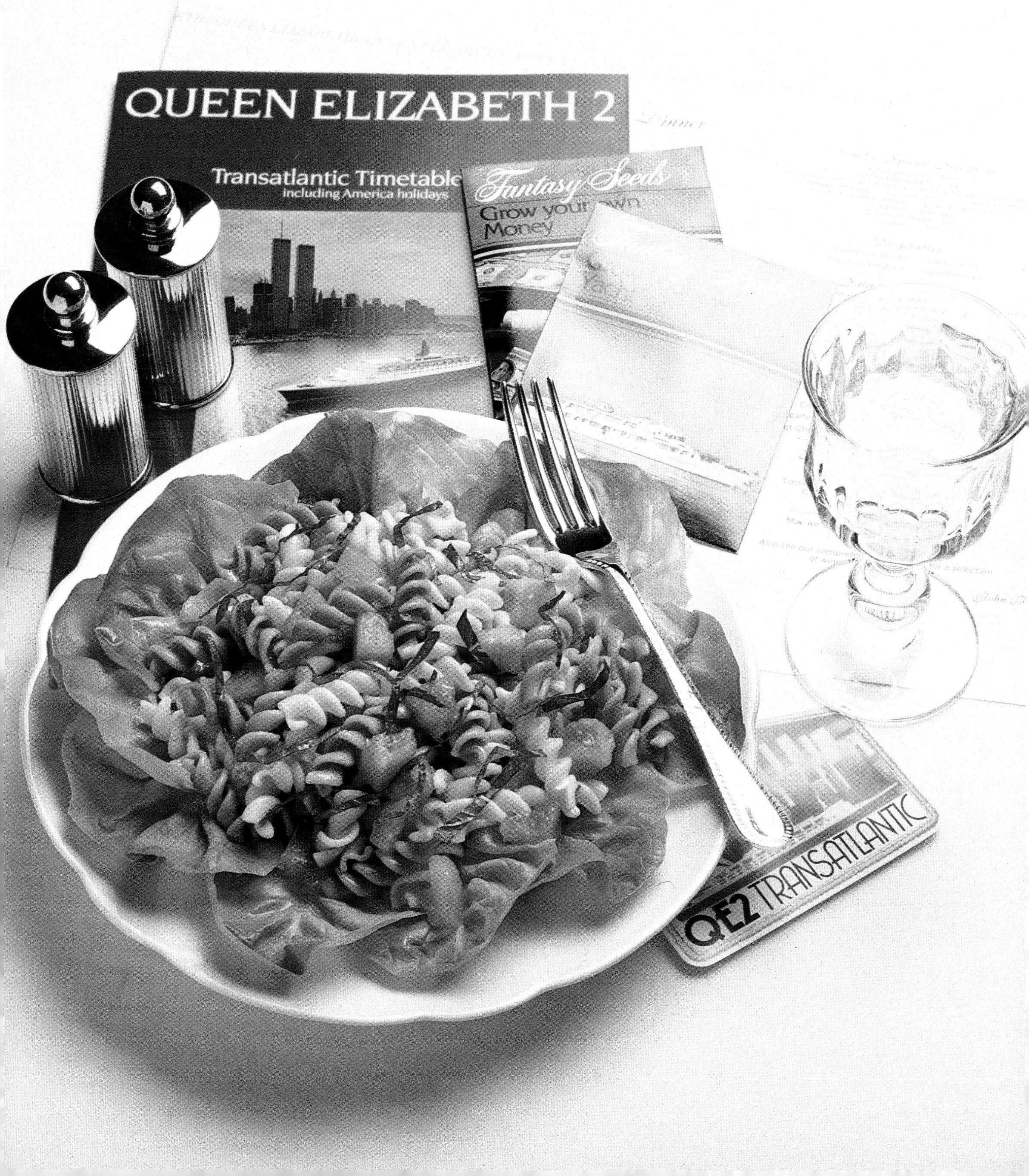
QUEEN ELIZABETH 2
Transatlantic Timetable
including America holidays
Fantasy Seeds
Grow your own
Money
QE2 TRANSATLANTIC

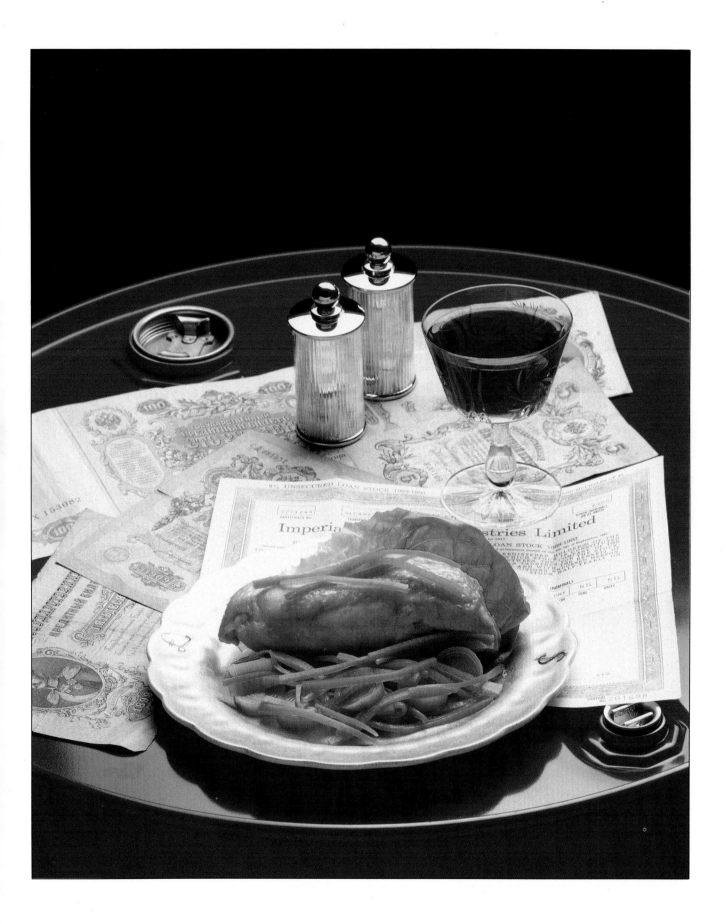

DINNER

> *Posh Poule au Pot*
> *Tomato and basil salad*
> *Fresh pineapple*

Posh Poule au Pot

The *en papillote* method of cooking fish in a foil or paper envelope also works frightfully well with chicken. Do not buy the average supermarket chicken if you can possibly avoid it, especially for use in a dish like this where the chicken is not disguised with a heavy sauce. Use either a free range or one of those bright yellow French maize-fed birds.

> *2 small carrots*
> *6 small leeks*
> *6 shallots*
> *oil*
> *2 chicken breast fillets of about 7 oz/200g each*
> *2 tbsp chicken stock*

Finely julienne the carrots, cut the white part of the leeks into ¼-inch/8-mm thick slices and chop the shallots. Take 2 large rectangles of aluminium foil and smear the centre of each with some oil. Put half the shallots on each piece of foil and a chicken breast on top of them. Place bundles of the julienne carrots around the chicken, and half the leeks on top of each piece of chicken. Moisten each breast with about 1 tablespoon of stock and then fold up the foil to make two packets. Put in an oven pre-heated to 400°F/200°C/Gas mark 6 and bake for about 30 minutes.

You can easily vary the vegetable contents of this tasty package by adding celery or some very thinly sliced mushrooms or some dried Italian porcini (which, of course, have first been soaked in tepid water for 45 minutes). This particular dish is amenable to endless variations and most vegetables – with obviously difficult-to-cook exceptions like potatoes, artichokes and aubergines – may be used in it. Instead of decanting the chicken and vegetables onto your plate, put the unopened packets on your plates and tear them open at the table for an appetizing blast of steam.

Tomato and basil salad is an excellent complement to this dish, which is quite robust, so you can serve any good middle range claret with it.

Follow with fresh pineapple and unsweetened tea or coffee.